Aging is *NOT* an Option!

10 9 8 7 6 5 4 3 2 1

The Baby Boomer's 10-Step Guide to a Long and Healthy Life

Andrew Keith

First Edition

Ageless Publications
P.O. Box 251544
Plano, TX 75025
www.agelesspublications.com

Distributor:
Wilson & Associates
P.O. Box 2569
Alvin, TX 77512 U.S.A.
www.thebookdistributor.com
E-mail: info@thebookdistributor.com
Phone: 281.388.0196
Fax: 413.683.8503

ISBN: 0-9741792-4-8
Library of Congress Cataloging Number: 2003112380

Book Design: Janice M. Phelps

PRINTED IN THE UNITED STATES OF AMERICA

Aging is *NOT* an Option!

In writing a book of this magnitude, it would never have come
to fruition if it weren't for the extreme understanding and help
of my wife. The many late nights and long days of work
squeezed in between raising children and other normal
commitments, the countless papers shoved in front of her face
asking her input or strongly suggesting that she read
and the numerous lifestyle changes we have gone through,
whether she liked them or not, I can never thank her enough.
I love you, honey.

To my kids who think that their dad is a health-nut . . .
well, I guess he is. Your mother and I plan on sticking around to
pester and embarrass you for a long, long time. So, get over it!

No animals were injured, euphemized, violated
or tickled incessantly during the production of this book.

Thank you.

Table of Contents

Disclaimer

This book is not intended to serve as a substitute for a physician, nor does the author intend to give medical advice. Readers are advised to consult their physician prior to embarking on any new health program.

Warning

America, this is your wake-up call! We, as a society, are getting fatter and lazier, are contracting many diseases at epidemic proportions, and, as a result, aren't living nearly as long as we should. We are in that proverbial "world of hurt" when it comes to our overall health. Even though we live in the greatest country in the world, our overall health is pitiful. In fact, The World Health Organization ranks us 37th in the world in the overall quality of health care! Surprised? Don't be. Even though we're living longer than our parents, we have made very little progress in finding cures for many of the life threatening diseases that we face such as heart disease, diabetes, and cancers, including colon, skin, breast, prostate and lung cancer.

The percentage of Americans classified as obese is increasing at horrendous rates. Richard Carmona, our U.S. Surgeon General, warned that we shouldn't lose sight of our biggest health threat, obesity. He called it an epidemic, saying that this totally preventable problem is killing 300,000 Americans annually. By age thirty-seven, 27% are considered obese and 34% are already overweight and on their way to the heavier classification. **Many studies estimate that two-thirds of all adult Americans are overweight.** We are becoming extremely sedentary and are getting less and less exercise, especially as we age, compounding the problem. Only 30% of us are working out on a regular basis and what's disturbing about is that it hasn't changed in several years.

Even our kids are getting into the act. Almost 20% of American children today are now considered fat. Sitting in front of a computer or television is becoming more the norm than the exception, compounding the problem. Not only are our schools wanting to remove physical education from our children's day, kids are taking prescription drugs more than they ever have. Out of the 53 million students in our country, more than 5 million of them are taking prescriptions for allergies, asthma, infections and, of course, attention deficit disorder. **The money spent on children's meds increased 28% in 2001 alone!** The number of American children taking psychiatric drugs has tripled since 1987, according to a study just released. Why the drastic increase? Why is it that American children consume 90% of the world's supply of Ritalin? We need to ask these questions. If they are obese and/or on prescription drugs now, what is going to happen to them after they become adults? Studies show that kids who are obese grow up to be adults with the same problems. **As healthy as *we* were as children, the decline of our respective health will be nothing compared to theirs.**

The corresponding results of our poor diet, lack of exercise and overall weight problem can be measured by the increasing number of ailments we are now seeing in our society. From obesity and lack of exercise, diabetes has raised its ugly head and is now running out of control. Over 16 million Americans presently have it and 2,100 new cases are diagnosed daily. That doesn't even include the millions of borderline diabetics that don't even have a clue that anything is wrong with them. As you probably know, diabetes will shorten your life, making you miserable before you expire. Adult-onset diabetes is not called that anymore. We didn't used to see this form of diabetes until its victims were in their forties or fifties. Not so anymore. Children as young as five-years old are now contracting this killer disease, which will shorten their now damned life anywhere from seventeen to twenty-seven years, according to a recent study. Because of the younger age affliction, it is now just called type-2 diabetes. That's a sad commentary on the state of today's health.

Colon, breast, cervical, lung and many other cancers are increasing at alarming rates. The same holds true for heart disease, Parkinson's, Alzheimer's and many other nervous system disorders. To further compound matters, our mental health system is in crisis. The number of Americans being treated for depression soared from 1.7 million in 1987 to over 6.3 million in 1997 and overall, our health care facilities are unable to provide even the most basic services and supports to those that need it. We may be living longer in general, but we are suffering more along the way. It doesn't need to be that way.

This is your wake-up call because if you are reading this, then you're probably a baby-boomer and your time on this rock is going to be more limited than you would like . . . unless you do something about it. If you are not taking *good* care of yourself, plenty of wonderful ailments and diseases are waiting for you right around the corner. Maybe a nice colon cancer or melanoma would suit you fine. How about a generous helping of high blood pressure? That could lead to a stroke or heart failure. How many of your friends or acquaintances already have been stricken with one of these? Is depression, kidney or liver failure, lung or breast cancer in your future? Don't forget about those nice little nervous system problems like Parkinson's, Alzheimer's or Lou Gehrig's diseases. There is a plethora of ailments that would love to make your acquaintance.

Fortunately, most of those are preventable. **In fact, the majority of all diseases are related to your specific environment and can be controlled or eliminated by an aggressive program used to improve your health.** In other words, don't smoke and you'll probably not get lung cancer. Improve your diet by eliminating fried, junk and processed foods and include fiber and nutritionally dense foods. Do these and your chance of getting colon cancer drops considerably. Lose the weight that you need to, and your risk of heart disease drops tremendously. The relative cause and effect relationship between your personal environment and disease has never been more pronounced than today.

This is serious business and can be life-threatening if you don't take it as such. There is hope, though. This program will give you most everything you need to improve the quality and length of your life. The ten steps outlined in this book cover all the major components of a well-rounded health program that will gear you towards a preventative lifestyle and put you on the road to an energetic, healthy and long life.

Premise

There have been many books written with the good intention of improving your overall health and well-being. I wouldn't even attempt to guess the number of books published trying to sell you on a certain type of diet, an exercise regime or a specific supplement to shove down your throat — herbs, machines, minerals or chemicals described as the proverbial fountain of youth.

Although many programs are worthwhile and would be of benefit if you were to use them, they all miss one crucial point, that being: **living long and in relatively good health is not about one specific item.** No exercise machine, herb, vegetable or drink is more than one piece of the overall puzzle. Put all those puzzle parts together, throw in several more, and then you may have something worth your time, commitment and effort. **One of the main premises of this program is that as you age, there are ten specific steps that must be followed in order to insure your good health and longevity.** Any one or two by themselves is incomplete and will only give you marginal results.

The nearest any plans come to offering a complete program are those that combine diet and exercise and then throw in a few other suggestions to round out what is defined as a thorough program. Still not enough. There are many more factors controlling your health than simply diet and exercise. One example would be getting the proper amount of restorative sleep. Without sufficient slumber, an exercise program won't do you much good. Ask any insomniac how they feel throughout the day and they will tell you that their days are usually very long and tiring. It doesn't really matter what they eat or how many miles they run, they are still miserable.

Do you usually get enough good quality sleep? Before you answer, think about the number of caffeinated drinks you need daily, or that lull that comes at about 4:00 in the afternoon. How about the tossing and turning or the snoring that you do at night? What about the effort it takes to pull yourself out of bed to shut off that blasted alarm that surely has gone off way too early? Has it taken the entire weekend to recharge your system from the previous five days of work? If you feel the need to improve your health, sleep is probably one area that you will want to work on. **It is imperative in any effective program that you rebuild and retool all of your body's cells that have sustained damaged from the day's activities.** Your brain also needs re-charging, and this is accomplished through the many steps taken during an uninterrupted good-night's sleep. If you don't get complete rest on a regular basis, the cellular damage inflicted will eventually get out of control, the end result being disease and illness. There have been countless studies showing the critical relationship between restful and restorative sleep and your overall health. **If you don't overcome any sleep problem that you have, your life will be shorter than you wish.** A consistent good night's rest is one of the ten steps outlined in this program, but remember that a good night's sleep is *still* only one of them.

During our teens and throughout our twenties, feeling good was easy. We were all Superman or Superwoman, even after a night to remember or, for that matter, several nights that weren't very easy to remember at all! (Come to think about it, can you remember any of them?) As we age, remaining healthy becomes more of a challenge and requires the contribution of many different facets, all of them working together to bring us where we would like to be in our lives. Ignore these many steps and your life will probably be over sooner than you would like.

There are ten steps needed to improve your overall health and that is our first premise. Each step will be thoroughly explained in its own chapter, backed by solid clinical research and studies.

Additionally, we must understand the evolution of the human body and how it has been designed to work and function properly. One of the obvious traits of humans has been our ability to survive. Many creatures have come and gone over the millions of years of this planet's existence, but man is still here. (Although we're trying really hard to blow each other up on a daily basis in an attempt to obliterate ourselves from the face of this planet.)

Why are we still here? Notwithstanding, our bent towards self-destruction, one of the primary reasons is our ability to adapt. If our ancestors weren't able to use what they had at their disposal and in their environment, we never would have made it to the present day. Millions of generations of change have fine-tuned our internal system to basically take care of itself. **This is the classic example of the biological law, "survival of the fittest."** Because of this fact of evolution, ***if given the chance, your body will heal itself.*** **This is the second premise of this program.** Whether it's the elimination of wastes, poisons and other unwanted substances through many complicated processes to the never ending battles that your immune system fights every second of every day, you were physiologically designed to take care of yourself.

You sometimes get a fever when you are ill, something no one enjoys. However, a rise in body temperature is one of the ways your system fights infection and disease. Even though it's not very comfortable, that mechanism is there for a reason, yet our first reaction is to get rid of it any way we can. Your body goes into overdrive in an attempt to rid itself of whatever is attacking it. Understand this self-preservation principle and learn how to give your body what it wants and needs in order for it to properly take care of itself. Instead of continually putting out fires, find out why the fires start in the first place. Embrace this philosophy and your chances of living a long and healthy life will increase tremendously.

Maybe the single most important aspect of this program and our third and last premise **is to put the control of your healthcare exactly where it needs to be, and that is with you.** ***You and only you should be controlling the direction of your life and your health.*** Not your doctor, not your family or friends, and certainly not your psychic or shrink. (Maybe your mother, though.) No one else knows what is good for you, except you (and your mother.) When you have control, when you are the one pushing the buttons, the results tend to be much better. Take your car to a mechanic and if something doesn't sound right in his analysis, then you go searching for another opinion: but have a health problem and you blindly follow the directions of your overworked doctor who may or may not know you or what you are going through. He may be able to take care of the problem and then again, he may not, for physicians are trained to look for pathology (disease) and then decide what pharmaceutical drug to prescribe. They know very little about preventative health, which could very well keep you out of their office in the first place.

Embrace the complete program described in this book, and you will increase your time on this planet. By following the ten steps outlined and using these three premises as your guide, your overall health will improve and the world will be a much better place for all of us to live in. When you're finished and on the road to a long and healthy life, join me in spending our children's inheritance and, while we're at it, let's break the social security fund!

Guarantee

Almost any health improvement program on the market today comes with some degree of a guarantee ranging from returning the product and refunding your money (good luck on that one!), to guaranteeing you profound health, the loss of half your body weight, an incredible body and/or beautiful looks. Not to be outdone, we would like to make you the following guarantee. The guarantee we are offering is that there is no guarantee in life. There is absolutely no guarantee concerning anything to do with you in life except the proverbial death and taxes. You may get run over by a semi-truck tomorrow, fall off a horse, run into a mass murderer, lose a limb, or never come back from the damage already done while in your younger, self-abusive days. Absolutely no one can predict precisely where you will be ten to twenty years from now, whether it concerns your career, your life and, until now, especially your health.

Take a trip into your neighborhood casino. (Almost every major community seems to have one.) Wander over to the blackjack table and ask the dealer to play a game with you. Take only one half of a deck of cards and make sure the ace of spades is included. Have the dealer shuffle them and then pick a single card. With half a deck you have a one in twenty-six chance of picking the ace of spades. Let's call that card the "black death" card. Pick it and you die. Ain't this fun! Take ten more cards out of the deck and your chances get much worse. Some of life is like this game. Most of us lead a life full of repetition. You walk out of your home, get into your car, go to work, come home, eat dinner and then go to sleep. Unfortunately your time can run out at any time, whether it's by horribly rotten chance, poor genetics, or just plain bad health. What if you begin with a full deck of cards instead of only half? Your chances become a lot better, don't they? How about adding another half deck (take the ace of spades out of that deck before adding). Now your chance of living is a whole lot better. Add more cards and your chances keep getting better. **That's what you'll be doing with this program — improving your chances for a healthy life.** Get back up to a full deck, or maybe add that extra half deck. (You've begun with that 26-card deck because of the way you have abused your body in the past.) Your warranty has been violated time and again and is now void with no chance of renewing. In fact, your warranty company won't even return your calls! "I didn't mean to do so much damage to the frame and the engine," you cry! Sorry, the man upstairs is about as deaf to that story as the IRS is with your reason for not filing your taxes for the last 17 years! Besides he know that he'll just get a chance to visit with you, in person, sooner. . .

Life is full of chances and your goal should be to stack the deck in your favor. Follow this program and you'll be adding cards faster and faster each step along the way. This is a great program and should increase your time on this planet's surface, not six feet under it.

Your life is also full of choices. Sometimes the choices that you make influence the chances of you living and dying. Take up cigarette smoking or skydiving and you lose a few of those cards. Begin eating too much and stop that exercise program and you lose several more. Lose too many cards and you won't have to worry about that freak accident like a freight train running off the tracks, down the hill and crashing into your bedroom while you sleep, killing you instantly. Make too many bad choices or not enough good ones and you may get lucky and die in your sleep, but however it happens, it will be sooner rather than later.

If you truly wish to get better, improve your health and live longer, then this program can certainly help. In fact, you will certainly feel and look better, have more energy and possess a better outlook on life in general by doing the things that are necessary and described in these pages. However, since no one can control drunken drivers, how well you follow this program or that crazy brother-in-law of yours, **the only true guarantees that can be given are from you and the man upstairs.**

This program is all about you taking control of your future. Not me, not your family and not your doctor. It's all about you grabbing that deck and adding several cards to it as often as you can. Then, you will be in control and that's the way it should be.

However, if it will make you feel better at this juncture, then of course, if you are not completely satisfied with this program, the publisher will reimburse the cost of this book. Are we square now?

Part 1:

Out of Control

Chapter 1:

Step Up to the Plate

Did you take your pill this morning? You know the one I'm talking about. The little pill that will make all of your troubles go away. The one advertised that will take twenty years off your life. How about the one that will give you the glowing skin tones of the supermodel shown holding that miracle in a bottle? Then there is the little white pill that will tone your muscles while you relax. The green one causing you to lose weight while you sleep (which you technically do anyway). What about the capsule that will give you the body of the Adonis in that magazine? Arthritis pain will be no more with this purple pill. Don't forget your sex life — that's the oblong one of course! Your cancer will be a distant memory and your mortgage will be paid off. Your kids will stop smarting off to you. Your luck will forever change. The beautiful people in your office, social circles, and neighborhood will now be jealous of you, your health and your good fortune. It's time to start playing the Lotto, for you will surely win now that you're taking that one tiny pill.

Sound familiar? Turn on your TV, especially on the weekends or late at night and you'll see countless infomercials touting the latest discovery that will turn your life around. There will be testimonials from people just like you bragging about how they "lost 650 pounds in just four months by taking this supplement." They say that you don't need to exercise or modify your life in any other way. Take the easy way; just take this capsule and you'll look like Heather Locklear, or Brad Pitt. God forbid if you have ever sent away for any health-related products, because you are now on ***that "one"*** mailing list. Congratulations, your mailbox will never be empty again! Just pull open the box and you will find the new you!

The distrust that the health-care and improvement industry causes in the presentation of their products is a sham *and* a shame. Some of it is, of course, junk. On the other hand many of the herbs, compounds and machines touted could really be beneficial to your health. **The problem is that they want you to believe that their product is *all* you need to look and feel wonderful, to turn back the hands of time . . . the proverbial fountain of youth in a can or bottle. The bottom line is this: There is no *one* pill, no one machine, no one product that will make all of your ills and maladies go away! There is not a pill in the world that can, or will, erase the thirty years of abuse that you have put your poor body through.** Even if you have taken relatively good care of yourself, good health is not about one particular item, pill, supplement, exercise or machine . . . it's a combination of many factors all working in unison, all having a purpose and a job to do, all contributing to your overall goal . . . good health. **The only way to extend your life and reach your full health potential this late in the game is by making a complete commitment towards that goal utilizing several different facets available to you.** Follow the ten-step program described in this book and you will not only feel better, you'll probably live longer. The next time you see one of those ads, just chuckle and remember that they exist only to sell you something.

Your good health is a combination of lifestyle changes and adjustments that you must embrace in order to change the way you look and feel. We'll cover the processes you need to implement in order to change the way you feel, give you some added energy, relieve some of your aches and pains, and hopefully add a few good quality years to the end of your life. Don't end up in a wheelchair unable to feed yourself, and don't wait until the last possible moment to begin afresh. **The longer you wait, the more difficult and less effective *any* program will be.** Will it be easy? Probably not; but that really depends upon your outlook, your disposition and how badly you want to make changes in order to enjoy life more. Look at *any* professional athlete. He probably doesn't enjoy all that he must go through in order to reach greatness. An athlete of that caliber has endured thousand of hours of preparation and sacrifice just to get to that one moment of success. Reaching the pinnacle of his career has made all of his toiling worthwhile. He had a goal and didn't waver from his aspirations for any reason. Neither should you.

Having good health and living long involves many different activities, habits, behaviors and maybe just a little bit of good luck along the way. Not coincidentally, all of your bodily functions, organs and systems all work together in synergy with the goal of achieving that "smooth running engine." better known as good health. It's imperative that you understand the symmetry involved among all of your body's functions, the interdependency that is required in order for you to run at your optimum efficiency.

Your lungs breathe in fresh air to nourish your entire system, and exhale much of the waste in the form of carbon dioxide. This oxygen-based mixture, of course, feeds your heart, which in turn pumps blood to every square inch of your body. The blood then returns bringing the waste with it to go through the cycle again, thousands of times a day. The nourishment that your liver just received allows it to do its job, which among other functions is to filter everything that enters your body. Lose your liver and your life ceases immediately. Poison your liver slowly and it will take its time killing you by trashing virtually every organ in your body and allowing all sorts of debilitating diseases to gain a foothold in your body. One of them will have the pleasure of finishing you off.

What happens if you decide to take up cigarettes? Besides wrecking your lungs, smoking slowly poisons the rest of your system by polluting its energy source, which is the clean, pure air that you are supposed to be breathing in. It should baffle you wondering why people purposely breathe smoke into their otherwise pristine lungs. However, cigarette smoking is too easy and obvious of an example. There are many more that may surprise you.

Take clinically diagnosed depression, as an example. Do you really think it's only a psychological disease? It can wreck havoc on the rest of your body, and in turn, affect the quality and length of your life. Depression has the ability to raise your blood pressure, destroy your immune system, contribute to osteoarthritis, osteoporosis, erectile dysfunction (not good!), complicate asthma and be a precursor to stroke. How could all of this happen just from some screwed-up brain chemistry? Why did this chemistry alter in the first place? Did you know that there is really no physical test for depression? No blood test, no EKG, no glandular exam, no x-ray or MRI, no SAT, PSAT, LSAT or even PB&J! So how is depression diagnosed? Believe it or not, it is diagnosed through its symptoms only; then those symptoms are treated through trial and error. Incredible as that sounds, unfortunately is the absolute truth. There is no test to positively identify it and on top of that, we rely on guesswork to treat it! Do you want someone guessing your ailment and then experimenting on you to try and control it?

Since traditional western medicine has no test for it, it isn't surprising that it doesn't know how to cure it either. The really unfortunate thing is that your doctor will never prescribe regular exercise, a change in diet, weight loss, or even sleep therapy . . . all of which can curb and maybe even cure depression. To think that all you have to do to control or cure depression is to hit the gym and the bed more and skip the dessert and happy hour bar is completely unheard of. We prefer some complicated diagnosis and pills to manage the problem instead. No wonder our bodies are so screwed up!

When you understand that your body parts and systems all work together in unison, then you'll be better able to control the quality of your life. Your brain is nothing more than a few pounds of chemicals and tissue that control the rest of your body, which in turn feeds and nourishes it, so it can do its job better. In fact, depression may not even begin in your mind. This mental illness may very well be a result of *other* chronic problems that you may have, though you may not relate them to brain chemistry. In this case, it's the proverbial "chicken or the egg" question. Did a long-term illness cause the depression or did the depression cause the other illness? Was it a lousy diet or poor lifestyle that preceded the depression? Why does physical or emotional trauma have the potential to screw up your brain chemistry? Hard questions to answer, but if you know the relationship between the different systems of your body, maybe you'll be better equipped to stop the breakdown before it even happens.

For as much as we do know, we still understand little about many organs and systems of our body, especially our brains. Our society has spent its collective time and efforts on electrical forms of energy, as in computers and automobiles. We have taken a computer the size of a Buick and made it a hundred times more powerful *and* shrunk it down to the size of a deck of cards. We can send people into space and back . . . yet we have no cure for depression. We really know little about how the human brain works or even why. There are all sorts of neurological disorders that all we have been able to do is to identify and maybe ease some symptoms. Break a computer or your car and we can fix them pronto. Fall and split your head open causing damage to your brain and most all we can do is to sit and wait . . . either you come out of it or you don't. Our lack of control in this area is amazing.

We are just beginning to understand what makes our body tick, and how to fine-tune it like you would a high-performance engine. Many of us are beginning to use common sense and are learning how to take care of our bodies in the form of preventative maintenance. For example, consider the composition of your brain. It is made up of nearly 85% water. Therefore, it only makes sense to replenish it on a regular basis with fresh pure water; not colas, not beer (sorry), not *Red Bull,* just plain, clean water. That makes sense, but seems to be too easy for us to comprehend. We're finally beginning to figure out that to feed our bodies the proper foods it needs, that maybe, just maybe, it might work better and perform longer. "That would also be too logical," Mr. Spock would say.

Years ago, you would have to take a fine car and occasionally "blow the carbon" out of it, which meant that it would have to be run hard and fast to clean the carbon buildup in the engine. (The detergent gasolines made today do that for us.) We humanoids need that too, only on a more regular basis. It's called exercise. Working out pumps blood much quicker than normal, helping to re-circulate the water supplying your brain. It stimulates the release of many different hormones, all of which are beneficial to the health of your personal think-tank.

Every function and every organ in your body are connected in some way. They all work together for your overall benefit. It seems like every day we get reports on studies that link a sedentary life and obesity with heart disease, diabetes and other ailments, yet seven out of ten American adults still do not exercise on a regular basis! That hasn't changed in several years. What are you waiting for? All it takes is four to five days a week of light to moderate exercises, which can include brisk walking for at least 30 minutes. That's fairly easy, yet we're too busy or lazy to get up off of our collective butts to extend our lives.

Did you know that constipated men are three times more likely to develop Parkinson's disease than men who aren't? Okay, stop laughing. It's not funny, especially to the ones suffering. People with semi-permanent corks up their . . . well, you know where, are at risk for Parkinson's. Incredibly, this relationship is true. This is a perfect example of what would seem like an off-the-wall relationship. Linking something at the south end of your body with the proper functioning of your brain may seem like a huge stretch, considering their relative locations, however the two can be related. A study published in *Neurology Magazine* tracked both men and women over a twenty-four-year time period showing a relationship between chronically constipated men and the incidence of Parkinson's (this particular study was inconclusive about a woman's risk). How is constipation related to a neurological disorder? Your intestinal system has several critical functions besides making sure that your waste speeds it way out of your body on a timely basis. If it stays around too long it can become very toxic. **Your exposure to toxins from any source can cause all sorts of neurological problems.** Parkinson's is only one of them. **Its other functions include manufacturing and releasing several different hormones, vitamins, minerals and enzymes to be used in the remainder of your system, including your brain.** Constipation inhibits all of these functions tremendously. It can be caused by stress, poor diet, not enough water consumption, lack of exercise and taking certain medications. These conditions are controllable by you. Every single one of these are critical areas that govern whether or not your entire system will remain healthy. Being constipated is nothing more than a symptom of your body performing at less than optimal standards, which can affect all areas of your health. Taking a pill is not the answer to constipation, nor to good health. Most medications are merely Band-Aids and do not correct the source of whatever the problem is. In this case, find out what is causing the stress to your system and correct the problem. **The constipation is only a symptom of bigger problems, and by taking a laxative you're not solving anything permanently.**

Another example is the relationship of periodontal disease and stroke. Recent studies have demonstrated that the same substance that sticks to your teeth causing certain gum disease also sticks to your blood vessels. This is yet another example of our body parts all working together. So, if you suffer from periodontal disease, it would be a good idea to monitor your cardiovascular system. **If you neglect one part of your body, others may crumble.**

As in the other aspects of your life, you must set goals when it comes to your health; however, they must be realistic. You may want to have several targets in mind because life is so full of variation. There is your family, your friends, your self-recognition and self-esteem. There is that closet full of clothes you cannot wear. How about the race you want to run? Golf, dances, grandkids, spouses, sex more than once every time a president is elected, energy and stamina. Maybe you're generally a grouch because you just don't feel good. Play catch with your kid, tennis with your spouse, and engage in many, many other activities you just don't do now because of a lack of energy.

Again, your goals need to be realistic, though. You're 40-, 50-, or 60-something and you're never going to win the Boston Marathon. You very well may run in one, and that by itself is a **huge** accomplishment. Go ahead and pat yourself on the back when you are finished, if you have the energy! Christie Brinkley is not in your future, neither dating nor looking like her. If you didn't have a great body as a kid, don't expect to resemble Arnold Schwarzenegger now. Don't set as a goal to be as skinny as Calista

Flockhart. That's probably not a healthy idea, anyway. Think of targets such as having more energy or getting your weight in the acceptable range for the next age group younger than yours! Why not live long enough to attend your grandchildren's graduation . . . from college! Stick around long enough to spend your kid's inheritance and to sufficiently spoil your grandkids. One of the best goals is to just feel good about yourself. Feel good about the way you look, about how you feel and your outlook on life in general. How about not being afraid to look at yourself in the mirror . . . naked!

Our knowledge of health and nutrition is easily tenfold our parents. We baby boomers gave birth to the running craze and the organic food movement, have seen several medical breakthroughs, legitimized acupuncture and chiropractic therapies, consumed tons of food supplements and even embraced Barry Manilow. We know so much more than mom and dad did about all forms of medicine and are beginning to get the picture on preventive care. **But for all of our advances, we seem to be ignoring most of what has become readily available to us in the name of laziness, and a strong lack of time management and conviction.** Look at yourself in the mirror and be truthful. How well have you taken care of that institution you call your body? Is it a temple, or a sleazy pool hall?

Step Up to the Plate

Do you truly want to improve your health and the length of your life? The obvious and quick answer is yes. Everyone does. **However, when it comes to making a commitment and taking action to improve your health, the vast majority of us pass on the opportunity.** Most of us don't really want to work for it. We don't have the time or patience in this instant gratification world of ours. If we don't see the results immediately then it obviously doesn't work. Maybe you won't do anything until you get one of those "wake up calls," like a heart attack. Sometimes that isn't even enough! Case in point: There was a study done on heart attack patients who were prescribed a specific and regular exercise program *after* their first attack **that would improve their chances of surviving another heart attack by a minimum of 25%.** Those seem like pretty good odds, especially when it comes to living or dying. In the beginning of this study, over 80% of the patients showed up for the program. (What possible excuse could the other 20% have had?) After only three years, the attendance was down to 13%. In other words, almost 90% of the people that had already had the proverbial "wake up call", an actual heart attack, apparently weren't interested in prolonging their lives enough to make the sacrifice needed to reach that goal and stave off another, probably fatal heart attack. **So, the question is, *"Do you really want to improve your quality of life?"*** Maybe you'll finish this book, and maybe you'll begin the steps necessary to delay Father Time, but will you stick with it until you get the call to go upstairs?

This program is not about a six-week, a six-month, or even a six-year effort. Although a six-year effort will do you a world of good, several months after you jump ship, you'll be back where you started. This program is about **you** gaining control of your life. It's about **you** seizing the opportunity to live longer and happier. No one, but **you** will govern **your** life for the next several decades. It is basically up to **you**. Hopefully **you** noticed the obvious overuse of the word "**you.**" It is not up to your doctor, brother, mother, husband, priest, lover, golfing partner, or your psychic. They could all be long gone by the time your story is finished. **This is something that you have to do for yourself and nobody else.**

The Prize Winners

Since the whole reason for this program is about extending your life and completing your journey in relatively good health, one question begs to be asked; "Is there any large sampling of people having success with this type of holistic approach about life and are they living longer, in general, that most other people?" (We're not talking about Joan Rivers. Stretching, tucking, folding and sucking can only go so far. Some day it's all going to snap and she'll be in three different counties!)

There are several pockets of communities all over the world that may not have all the modern conveniences that we in America have come to enjoy and expect, like pizza delivery, and most of them don't have the degree of healthcare available that we do, but still they live a longer and healthier life than Americans. It's difficult to accurately document some of the communities, especially the ones inhabiting far off and remote areas of our rock we call Earth, so coming to absolute conclusions about the benefits of their lifestyle may be a stretch.

However, there is one entire island of homo-sapiens that has done a wonderful job of preserving themselves and enjoy much better health than we do. You may have recently read about the Okinawans and the research done on them called "The Okinawa Program." Although the name that the researchers picked for their study sounds rather boring and may lull you to sleep, their findings are just short of amazing. **Okinawans have the longest disability-free life expectancy in the entire world!** More of their people live to be over one hundred than anywhere and most of their elderly live independently, not in nursing homes. They have 80% fewer heart attacks than Americans, and the ones that do are more likely to survive than here in the states. Most cancers, especially breast and prostate are rare among Okinawans, and the normal markers of old age like dementia and cardiovascular disease are equally as infrequent. In general, there is no obesity on the island (other than an occasional visit by Anna Nicole Smith) and they will probably live seven to ten years longer than you.

So what the heck are they doing and can we bottle their

drinking water? The answer is simple on one hand, but on the other hand it is not. No, you cannot bottle their water. That's the simple part. **What makes them successful is that they have a complete lifestyle, not just a single behavior that they practice that gives them the top health award on this planet.** There is not just a certain fish or plant that they consume, nor is there one philosophy they employ that causes them to live so long. The only factors different than us that may contribute to their longevity is that they have no chicken-fried-steak, MTV or Barney. Other than that, they breathe the same air, have the same number of arms and legs, and exercise the same power of choice that we Americans do.

It's their **choices** that are the main difference. They choose to eat healthier, choose to be more active for a longer time and choose not to let stress get the better of them. You'll notice that, like you, they still have stress. After all, they have children, don't they? They just elect to handle parenting differently. (I believe they eat their young.)

What's their secret, or more aptly, secrets? First, their diet is much different than ours. You could have guessed that, though. To start, they consume an average of seven servings of vegetables daily. Well, we just lost the majority of you who think that there is no way you are going to come close to eating that many servings of peas and okra daily! (Relax; donuts are made with vegetable oil, so they qualify. That should make you feel better . . . not!) You don't necessarily have to duplicate their lifestyle to get some of the health benefits enjoyed by them. They also consume several servings of grains, like noodles, rice, of course, and bread everyday. That sounds more doable, doesn't it? Next, they have two to four daily servings of fruit, lots of soy products, green fish and tea . . . or is that green tea and fish? Take your pick. Bean sprouts, sweet potatoes, onions and seaweed are some of the most prominent staples of their diet. (Don't rush out and buy a ton of seaweed, now!)

Using weight as a gauge, vegetables, grains and fruit make up over 70% of their diet, soy and that seaweed make up another 14%, fish about 11%, and the "biggie" fact here is that meat, poultry, and eggs account for only 3% of what they eat. They stay away from the foods highest in fat and cholesterol. Of those, chicken is probably eaten most. (If chicken is not available, they just search for neighborhood cats or dogs...only the young ones, though.)

They also put an emphasis on dark green vegetables that have a lot of calcium. They get much of their required protein from fish and soy, and they stay away from the simple sugars found in so many of our processed foods. They concentrate their palates on complex carbohydrates that do not spike their blood sugar levels and thus the main reason that diabetes is very uncommon among Okinawans.

They don't sit around watching *Jerry Springer* all day, either. Spending time on martial arts (even the much older Islanders), gardening, walking, and manual labor for their entire lives has been ingrained in them for generations. So another one of the keys to their longevity is that they stay active. It probably doesn't matter what they do, just that they do something that involves working their bodies.

They drink alcohol, just not very much. They are a very spiritual people and hold their women in high esteem within their culture. Let's not take that point lightly. There are many parts of this world where women are considered inferior to men, adversely impacting at least half of the population, if not all of them.

Although this program is not patterned after the Okinawan study (it came out in the middle of writing this book), their lives are certainly worth observing. Duplicating the lifestyle of the Okinawans may be tough, but taking some of their principles to heart may buy you some extra years on this planet. Cut down on your meats and junk foods, processed foods, get off your butt and do some sort of exercise and having some spirituality can help a whole lot. Meditating and chanting on your bus ride to work isn't necessary, although that might keep the nuts and petty criminals away from you! And if you are out of chicken, please don't harm any neighborhood pets, unless they're young and tender!

Chapter 2:

Fat Boy's

I recently passed a fireworks stand that went by the name of Fat Boy's Fireworks. Now that's someone comfortable with himself! "Yeah, I'm fat. Do you want cherry bombs or M-80s?"

Since there is a ton of data on obesity coming out as this program is being committed to paper (or more correctly, the computer), it is appropriate to give the subject of being overweight its own hefty chapter. As with smoking, drug addiction and criticizing your spouse, being obese is another "lifestyle choice" that will not only shorten your life, but will make the journey there a lot more difficult. Breathing smoke into your lungs doesn't even *sound* like it makes much sense. Injecting heroine into your arm is just plain stupid. Telling your wife that she isn't pretty is even worse. But eating that piece of pie doesn't sound like much of an offense. It looks good, your mouth is salivating and your brain tells you that you need this tiny piece of sweetness. After all, your mother made it especially for you, didn't she? After eating that little piece of heaven, the brain chemicals produced made you feel wonderful, confirming your choice. That's tough to resist. One of the problems with taking in excess calories is that they add up rather subtly. A little here and a little there can sneak up on you and before you know it your mid-section enters a room before you. One hundred calories daily isn't much and amounts to about one-half of a medium-sized candy bar. If you can eliminate that alone from your diet, you'll save 35,000 calories in a year. That's ten pounds!

"Are **you** fat?" That was probably not a politically correct question to ask. Aren't we supposed to have compassion for "people of size"? After all, they're just like you and I; there's just more of them, as in "more weight being carried by each of them" as opposed to "more of them in this country." Unfortunately, both statements are becoming truer every day. Fat people obviously weigh more, *and* **according to the Center for Disease Control, obesity is swiftly becoming the leading cause of preventable death and illness in the U.S. The key word here is preventable. It is vaulting ahead of smoking as the number one avoidable "trip to the other side."** Pretty soon, thin and fit people will be the minority and America will not be "inherited by the meek," but overrun by the plentiful.

"The second day of a diet is always easier than the first. By the second day, you're off it." –Jackie Gleason

This is not a worldwide problem, though. The United States of America, the most powerful country in the world, the most developed, the best educated, has the most advanced society, and arguably contains the highest number of intelligent people on this planet; so why are we ranked 12th out of the thirteen industrialized nations in the world in terms of health indicators such as infant mortality and life expectancy? On top of that wonderful distinction, the World Health Organization ranked us 37th in overall healthcare as a nation. Don't they have any respect for the greatest county in the world? I guess not. Get rid of smoking and obesity and I'd be willing to bet that we would gain at least some ground on the rest of the world when it comes to health issues. However, that doesn't cure our pathetically high percentage of uninsured citizens nor our failing health and lack of preventative care, but that's another battle to be covered later. So lose the cigarettes and the excess baggage (not your spouse!), if not for yourself, for the sake of America!

Today, about 300,000 Americans die from illnesses attributed to obesity annually. That's more than we lost in any recent war and at least as many as from cigarettes. As far as smokers are concerned, they have now been diminished to being considered second-class citizens. They are forbidden from partaking in a perfectly legal activity from restaurants, busses, planes, public places, government buildings, bathrooms and even public parks . . . outside. Legal that it may be and as deadly as it has become, obesity is swiftly passing it up as the numero uno cause of avoidable death.

Sixty-five percent of all adults and at least 15% of all children are fat, and the percentages are getting worse. Some even put the adult figure closer to 70%! In the last twenty years, the number of teenagers considered obese has tripled! Not surprisingly, the onset of type 2 diabetes has multiplied tenfold since the '80s. Of adult Americans born between 1957 and 1964, 34% are already considered obese and 35% are just overweight and heading for that bigger classification. Each decade, we get more sedentary, put on more weight and suffer from more ailments. It's not surprising since we consume more and more processed foods each and every year. **In fact, we are consuming 500 more calories a day than our society did back in the 1950s; most of it in the form of refined grain products, added sugars and fats.** I guess it's just pure coincidence that as we get fatter, we have more disease and illnesses, our prescription and hospitalization costs go up and we lose more days in bed than before? Hmm . . . maybe not.

"My doctor told me to stop having intimate dinners for four, unless there are three other people there." –Orson Welles

Who is to blame and what are the risks? Obesity is more costly, more deadly and, in the long run, much more painful than smoking, drinking **and** reckless driving. It does, however, allow you to get more for your money when you shop for clothing, assuming you can get clothes to fit. A size six generally costs the same as a sixteen. How about the "all you can eat" buffets? You can really get your money's worth if you try. It took me a long time before I could go into one of those restaurants and not go back for seconds and thirds. Had to get full value out of the trip there. Those places are not a problem for me anymore. I just stop at Krispy Kremes before I hitting the buffet! Takes care of **that** little problem!

Does anybody die from obesity? There is generally no classification of "obesity" on the average death certificate, even though there should be. Just like smoking, people merely die from all of the diseases that obesity causes, like diabetes; heart, liver and kidney disease; hypertension and strokes. Being fat is also similar to stress in that it goes undiagnosed, has no one specific cause and induces failure of your immune system and many organs, while taxing the hell out of your entire body. The only difference is that you can't see stress.

It surely causes, or at least helps the onset of arthritis, which adds pain as another characteristic of being fat. Your body wasn't built or meant to carry excess weight on its frame. Your heart doesn't have the capacity to pump the amount of blood needed to properly supply your limbs and organs when you have too much bulk. On top of that, fat cells, although a small number are needed for emergencies, are not very efficient in design. They don't have the blood capillaries necessary to carry blood to and waste away from your cells. They are literally just "a blob" of "goo" plastered to your midsection, chin, thighs, face, arms and of course your belly.

Anyone care for a hip replacement? How about a new knee? Note: recently there was a product recall that you may remember. A company that manufactures artificial hips was forced to recall their defective product! Ouch! How does that work? How do you recall a bad artificial hip? I can't imagine *one* surgery, let alone another to remove the defective hip and replace it with hopefully a better one!

Diabetes is up nearly 50% in the past decade. Obesity is almost synonymous with diabetes. **The number of Americans having this ailment is quickly approaching 20 million, some of them not even realizing that they are nearing this debilitating milestone. The American Diabetes Association predicts that one million more Americans will be diagnosed every year,** and the unfortunate part of this equation is that once you get diabetes you generally can't get rid of it. This monster will kill you by starving your organs . . . slowly.

The number one pre-cursor of diabetes is obesity. Gain only eleven extra pounds and you double your risk of catching diabetes. 82,000 amputations annually are done because of diabetes. Being considered obese quadruples your risk of getting diabetes. Do you like to read? The number one cause of blindness is diabetes. It plays havoc on your blood-sugar levels and adversely affects any organ that require a concentration of oxygen like your heart, liver and eyes…

Even our kids are getting in the act. Type 2 diabetes (the one that obesity causes) used to be known as "adult-onset diabetes." They don't call it that any more. Children as young as five-years-old are contracting diabetes and 80% of them are obese! Contracting diabetes at such a young age will shorten their lives up to twenty-seven years, according to a recent study. **The bottom**

line is that if you are fat, you greatly increase you chances of contracting diabetes and dying sooner than necessary. That can't be stated any simpler or more direct . . .

"Life expectancy would grow by leaps and bounds if green vegetables smelled as good as bacon." –Doug Larson. (Amen, brother!)

Back to the original question: Who is to blame? Should we have compassion for heavy people? Let's look at smokers in comparison. Personally speaking, I don't dislike smokers, nor am I insulted by their behavior. Even though it is one of the worst habits anyone can have, I feel sorry for the social stigma that follows them. They are not breaking any laws and are already being punished by the taxes added to the cost of a pack of cigarettes. They will suffer enough later in life without us adding to their addiction problem.

Caring for the health of a smoker is another issue, though. Should you and I have to finance the cost of taking care of smokers? Oh yes, there are plenty of extra costs that *someone* has to pay for. Smokers eventually spend a whole lot more time in the hospital and in convalescent care than non-smokers. Their costs in lung disease, missed work, heart attacks, and several different types of cancers are huge. Who pays for the billions and billions of extra, unnecessary costs? We, the taxpayers of the United States do, of course. I don't like it and I am guessing that neither do you. In fact, several recent surveys showed that most Americans don't like it either. Making a decision to smoke is just that. It is a conscious deliberate decision of going to the vending machine, plucking down $4 in quarters, finding some matches and then lighting up just so that they can breathe smoke into their lungs.

I'm sure that most of us non-smokers don't understand the addiction part of the equation, but that is not our problem, and for that matter isn't the problem of the cigarette companies. It is a legal substance with plenty of warnings plastered on the packages. (By the way, what happened to all of the money the states wrangled out of the cigarette companies? Wasn't it supposed to take care of the people directly affected by smoking?) There is a huge hypocrisy in dealing with the issue of holding the cigarette companies accountable. All of the money received by the states seems to have gone to a few attorneys and into the states' general funds, but very little, if any, to the smokers or family of the smokers. What sense does that make? The obvious answer is to make cigarettes illegal, but I don't think that will happen anytime soon.

Back to the original issue of obesity. Should there be a warning placed on a package of potato chips? Why the warning on a pack of cigs and not on that bag of chips? Obesity raises an individual's health-care costs by 36% and medication costs by 77%, much farther than from tobacco or drinking.

Should the restaurant industry be held accountable? Aren't they the ones pushing the "biggie-size" servings, the sixty-four-ounce colas, the sixty-four-ounce steaks, the chicken fried steak smothered in gravy? Mmmm, makes me hungry thinking about it! Did you know that the average-sized restaurant dinner plate was ten inches in diameter just a decade ago? Today, in order to accommodate the huge portion sizes, the average is now twelve to thirteen inches! Let's blame their ad agency or the National Restaurant Association. Maybe they should have to pay. Surely you and I are not to blame. After all, isn't the restaurant industry forcing the bigger portions on us? Do they actually expect us to have self-control? Come on, if we don't eat the food, someone else will. Pass the bread sticks, please.

Well, at least let us blame the fast-food portion of the restaurant world. In the early days of fast food, hamburgers, french-fries and drinks were all smaller than they are today. It seems to me that they have all conspired to get us hooked on their food product and then began increasing portion sizes until we are consuming, in one meal, what many poor Asian people eat in 30 days. Fat, fat, fat, sugar, sugar and more sugar. Give it to them until they get hooked. In the meantime, we (the evil restaurant CEOs), will invest in the health-care industry, and then we'll have all of the money!

What about your local PTA groups? They are forever having candy sales in schools and on the streets. That's a great example for our kids, isn't it? Let's train them from an early age that it's okay to reach for that Snicker's bar when hungry. That doesn't make a lot of sense either. Our school systems enter into very lucrative contracts with soft drink companies to put vending machines stocked with sugar-laden drinks down every school hallway. Some think that is a sell-out, damning our children's health in the name of profitability and budgets. I don't disagree.

"I'm at the age where food has taken the place of sex in my life. In fact, I've just had a mirror put over my kitchen table."
–Rodney Dangerfield

Early grocery stores consisted mainly of produce, fresh meats and a fresh bakery. I would be willing to bet that those sections make up a very small minority of the total square footage in today's supermarket. It should be the opposite.

You will never get your weight where it needs to be if you depend upon the restaurant industry or processed foods for the bulk (pardon the pun) of your diet.

What do **you** think? If you're one of the "weight-challenged" folks, then probably not much, right about now. You're probably getting steamed at this point. If you're carrying too much weight and are insulted by this, sorry, it wasn't meant to be demeaning. I have several good friends and family members that are heavy, and I have as much compassion and love for them as I do for anybody.

It's just that they probably won't live as comfortably nor as long as they could if they were not obese, and that is a shame. Does anybody wish for people to suffer more than they should have to and leave this planet sooner than necessary? Of course not. Especially when ***they*** really control that part of their own destiny! For the most part, they do not have to be heavy. No one is in control but themselves. If there is any addiction involved, then it certainly isn't as severe as a tobacco addiction. God doesn't control their weight, nor genetics for the most part, nor their family, their job, and certainly not any fast food restaurant. Life didn't hand them a bad deck of cards. In fact, we all have pretty much identical decks, the same pressures, the same twenty-four hour clock and the same food industry.

I don't know you and probably will never meet you, so what you do with your life is totally up to you. It's none of my business, nor should it be anybody else's, for that matter. And to answer that question above, personally I have plenty of compassion for the people in my life regardless of how they look. I'm not so sure the rest of this country mirrors that sentiment, though. Several surveys out seem to point to America's lack of compassion for the "weight-challenged" person. Again, with obesity, the issue is of control; **your** control over **your** life. **Your** hand is on the trigger, on the remote and on your future. After all, we do live in America, the land of the "free to do whatever the hell we want," just as long as we pay our taxes, of course!

On the other hand, since being overweight greatly hinders your health, I personally would love nothing more than to see this program do wonders for you. It would be wonderful for your life to be extended, for it to be much more comfortable, for you to bound out of bed in the morning ready to take on the world and maybe put a smile on your face a little more often. Walk up that flight of stairs with your friends and watch them struggle while you're just grinning from ear to ear. I can't think of a better compliment or a more worthwhile feeling than to know that this program made a marked difference in you life. If you have a lot of weight to lose and this program helps you accomplish that, then great! Maybe Jarred from Subway is who inspires you; that's fine too. Just be inspired.

I know plenty of chubby kids that grew up to be skinny adults. I also know skinny kids that . . . well let's say that they "blossomed" when they became adults and now have to turn sideways to get through a doorway. Same lives, same choices, same circumstances. What happened to them and their lives? Nobody knows but them. What we do know is that it wasn't genetics that made them heavy, which basically means that genetics can't be used as an excuse. Oh, their parents may have influenced how they look, but it was more of a behavioral pattern taught at the dinner table that they passed on, rather than genetics. **Genes control your height, the color of your eyes and whether or not you are going to be bald, but it does not control how much you eat and then as a result how much you weight.** Mother Nature doesn't have it out for you. She may punish you more than others if you get off the bandwagon for too long, but you control the way you look and, for the most part, the way you feel.

WHY DOES FAT MATTER?

There are dozens of reasons why your health is crucially dependant upon how much you weigh, so as not to bore you, we'll concentrate on the **top ten reasons** that you should be concerned about your size. You'll see that "the top ten reasons" will be a recurring theme in this book due to its simplicity, its ability to help you remember things and because David Letterman uses it . . . come to think of it, do I need his permission? I hope not because he may be difficult to reach. Anybody have his phone number?

The Top Ten Reasons to Shed that Spare Tire

1. **To Prevent a Heart Attack.** Being obese raises the risk of heart disease at least 50% by itself! Between two and three million Americans suffer from heart attacks annually. By placing too much pressure on your heart to perform more than it was intended causes your most important organ (even more important than the male penis) to give out and fail (kind of like an old penis). As you probably know, open heart surgery, involves sawing your chest wide open with a Sears-brand skill saw, then breaking every one of your ribs while peeling back the protective cage just to get to your ailing heart. That's even before doing any work on the old clunker! That doesn't sound like a whole lot of fun. Getting your weight down to where it needs to be will give your heart a break. Permanently filling the back end of your car with heavily-weighted sandbags will kill your engine in the same way that carrying excess weight will total your heart.
2. **To Prevent Diabetes.** You become fat because you have consumed more calories that your body needs, to put it simply. Most of those calories do a wonderful job of spiking your blood sugar level too quickly, forcing your pancreas to pump out more insulin to compensate. Eventually, like your heart, your pancreas will give out. That's when your life turns into an utter hell. Diabetes puts a tremendous strain on your body at the cellular level (the cells of your body, not your cell phone), eventually killing them, and in turn decimating your organs. Diabetes is the leading cause of adult blindness, limb loss, heart attack and many cancers. Don't even think of a pancreas transplant . . . it hasn't been done yet. Being obese is, by far, the number one factor in contracting diabetes.
3. **To Prevent Strokes and Hypertension.** Too much pressure on the walls of your blood vessels can cause a world of problems

including stroke and all sorts of different heart and circulatory diseases. Strokes are a consequence of a loss of blood flow to your brain, killing off brain cells in whatever portion of your brain it occurred in. A stroke can be caused by either a blood clot or a bursting of the vessels carrying the blood to your brain, both cutting off the flow of oxygen where it is needed for life. You have seen people that have had strokes . . . it's not very pretty. Besides, you don't want people to see you drool all over yourself, do you? Being heavy can cause increased blood pressure. Unfortunately, suffering from a stroke can be very permanent, something you don't want.

4. **To Prevent Arthritis.** Obesity greatly increases the possibility of contracting one or more of the many forms of arthritis. Arthritis, which is an inflammation and deterioration of your joints, happens, in part, when your joints cannot handle the amount of pressure placed on them. Live your life on a space station where there is weightlessness and arthritis doesn't happen. Unfortunately not too many of us are going to have that chance. Less weight means less physical stress at the intersection of two bones. That translates into less deterioration of your joints. Excess weight causes a "design flaw" in the equipment, for you engineering geeks. Your body was made to carry only so much weight. Exceed the limits and you void your warranty.
5. **To Reduce Free Radical Production.** Free radicals are molecules considered unstable because they are missing electrons. They apparently feel guilty about that missing electron, causing them to break the law and "steal" one from another otherwise healthy molecule, turning that molecule into a free radical itself, making it defective. When your body's defense mechanism (including antioxidants) fails to eliminate these rogue invaders, the process causes an adverse chain reaction throughout your body, causing damage at the cellular level in the beginning, while the ultimate long-term effect means premature death. Almost all illnesses in the human body are

caused, in the beginning, by free radical damage. This next point is very important to understand. The creation of free radicals happens every single time you put food in your mouth. It is a natural bi-product of your digestive process, similar to automotive emissions. So, by eating less, you lessen the occurrence of free radicals in your system allowing your disease fighters more of an opportunity to do their job. (This isn't the only way free radicals are formed, but nonetheless is one method that you have some control over.)

You don't want your immune system to get literally overwhelmed by an onslaught of free radicals. Can you say "General George Custer"? It has been proven clinically that if you reduce your daily calorie consumption you will live longer. As an example, take a normal 2000-calorie-a-day diet and reduce it to 1400–1500 permanently and you will see more birthdays. (The substitution has to be of nutritionally dense foods, though, not junk.) In fact, this is the only longevity practice that has actually been proven in a laboratory. Eat less — live longer.

6. **To Reduce Your Health-care Costs.** Obesity is not healthy and has been shown to cost a lot more in health-care over a lifetime; so by losing weight, you will spend less time in front of a doctor, in a hospital, off of work and free of costly medication. Of course you may then spend all of your spare time and newfound energy at the racetrack blowing a small fortune on some distant cousin of Seattle Slew, but hey, what the heck. At least give your money to someone you want to instead of the health-care industry. Again, make it entirely your choice.
7. **To Prevent Cancers.** This oftentimes fatal classification of disease is usually caused by molecules "run amuck," better known as free radicals. The less free radicals, the less chance of becoming ill with cancers of all types. Cancer cells require more sugar to survive, excess sugar consumption causes *more* fat, so having *less* fat will help starve them off, too. Take better care of yourself by eating better foods, and dining less often and you will supercharge your immune system, which will

thank you by doing battle with all the little Gremlins that wish to do you harm.

8. **It will be easier to improve your health in other ways.** Exercise becomes easier with less weight to carry around. You can walk and jog further and with less effort. Because of the pains you took in losing your excess weight you will be more inclined to watch what you eat. Sleep, a huge factor in your overall health, will be less of a problem. In short, becoming healthier will be a lot simpler with less weight.

9. **You will look and feel better.** I'm sure you're familiar with those amusement park mirrors that make you look like Roseanne. Do all the mirrors that you gaze into reflect that same look? Lose the spare tire and you will look and feel better and, most importantly, you will feel better about yourself.

10. **To Lower Food Costs.** Most people think that junk food is generally cheaper than nutritionally dense foods (that would be foods that actually give you some nutritional benefits). In some cases, yes, that is true. A candy bar may be cheaper or more readily available than an apple or banana. As far as meals go, however, it's a lot less expensive to consume healthier foods than the proverbial steak-and-potatoes American diet. Make a huge salad with all sorts of good, natural and healthy fruits, vegetables, nuts and beans. Eat all you wish and throw out the rest, and you probably still spent less than on a good steak or casserole. Beans are cheap; nuts in moderation are the same. A small, lean piece of chicken or fish broiled, baked or grilled isn't that costly. Steam some vegetables, eat low-fat yogurt for breakfast, make a big pot of soup and use long grain rice or good pasta for filler, and you haven't spent very much. Hell, you can make an entire meal around a baked sweet potato! Granted, it's not as easy as picking up a breakfast bar, but eating properly pays huge dividends . . . for less money spent.

"All the mistakes I ever made were when I wanted to say ' No' and said 'yes' instead." –Moss Hart

You be the judge

Let's get back to the original questions posed in the beginning of this section: Are you fat? How do you objectively decide whether you are a normal size or not? How do you know if you are running an increased risk of heart disease? Are you going to end up with diabetes? What's your favorite color? Just curious. **If you are fat, obese or whatever you wish to call it, the percentages go way up when you talk about life-threatening diseases. Gain just a few pounds and your risk of heart attack can double! Cold hard facts, studies and clinical observations show time and time again that being overweight will shorten your life and very easily make you miserable before you get to the end.**

If you are really interested in knowing where you are presently in this game of attempting to live longer, then you have to have some way to measure your level of fitness, as far as weight is concerned. You're either fat or you aren't. Okay, maybe some of us are in between.

The simplest way to tell is just to remove all of your clothing and stand in front of a mirror . . . yes, naked. No, not the one at Macy's! You may want to take this test in the privacy of your home and make sure that when you faint, that there is carpeting underneath you. Don't ask your spouse if you are fat. They didn't end up staying married to you this long by being stupid! "No dear, you're not fat. I love you just the way you are" is the only answer that you're going to get.

It's test time

What if you don't feel that you look bad, especially for your age? After all, most of your friends don't look as fit as you. Well, you may not be overweight, but just to be sure, science has devised some wonderful charts, graphs, and formulas to help you figure it out. Ross Perot would be proud.

One judge is the **Body Mass Index** or **B.M.I.** It sounds like some Ivy league school or a type of Wall Street analysis, doesn't it? You can figure your B.M.I. by using the following simple equation: divide your weight by your height in inches. (No cheating!) Divide that figure by your height in inches again and then multiply that figure by 703. Don't ask me how someone came up with that formula, but it is pretty well accepted as a good indicator of where you stack up, no pun intended. If your answer was less than twenty-five, then congratulations are in order. You can eat that banana split! A tally of twenty-five to thirty is considered overweight and the grand prize for a score of over thirty is obesity and a shorter life.

Now before you have a heart attack because your overgrown muscles or large body frame put you over and you feel you're in pretty good shape, this doesn't work for everyone. Emmitt Smith, I'm sure, is over thirty on this scale . . . you can tell him that he is fat, because I'm not going to be the one! If you're 5'10" and 220 pounds of muscle, then this system won't work for you. Being "big-boned" may not apply either.

You more than likely will need more than one measurement to judge whether on not to start that diet. The next measurement that is very useful is to measure your percentage of body fat. You can do that several different ways. The first involves being submerged in water using fairly sophisticated equipment and probably isn't an option for most of us. It's the most accurate method, but it's not really necessary at this point. All that you really want to do is to get a general idea where you are on the "fat" scale. The next method, which utilizes a handheld electronic reader, is too general, though, and you shouldn't trust the readings. There's no way that a piece of equipment that measures just your hands and then imputing your body weight can accurately measure your body fat.

The most practical method is to be measured by someone that is knowledgeable, like a fitness trainer or physical therapist, using calipers to "pinch" you in specific parts of your body, then compiling the readings together to figure your percentage of body fat. They can measure as little as three locations and as many as ten or eleven, depending upon their guidelines. I believe that the more pinch points, the better. Do this a couple of different times using the same person and the same calipers and you'll get a more accurate reading. This particular method has been around for years and still yields the easiest and best readings.

THE GRADING SCALE

The range of body fat allowed to be considered healthy is way too lenient, but here are the ranges nonetheless. If you are between forty and fifty-nine (that's age, not body fat percentage), you are considered healthy if your percentage of body fat is between 23–33% for women and 11–21% for men. Just another example of discrimination against men! Women get to eat more cheeseburgers than men . . . not fair. If your age falls between sixty and sixty-nine, you get 24–35% fat if you're a woman and 13–24% for men. Again, not fair. Anything over those numbers and your eulogy will be sooner than desired. Again, I feel that the numbers are too high. Men should certainly be under twenty percent and women less than thirty, but they didn't ask me for my opinion. That hurt my feelings . . .

There's one last benchmark and that is the ratio between your waist and hips. It's a fairly new measurement, but good to use to measure your overall health. The reason being that fat that is the most dangerous to your health is the kind that shoves your waist out in front of you. If you exercise on a regular basis, you'll get rid of a lot of that, thus making you healthier. To calculate, measure your waist at the narrowest point (if you have one) and your hips at the widest (not difficult to find). Divide the waist reading by the hip. Make sure and not reverse the equation! Your goal should be a number under 0.92. In other words, your waist should be smaller than your hips as in Dolly Parton, not W.C.

Fields. Oops! Sorry about that; please don't shoot the messenger! That's what this program is for. It will help bring those measurements down, if you give it a chance.

Scare tactics

I'm not above scaring the hell out of you in order to get you to follow the steps outlined in this program. America needs a wake up call anyway. Sometimes reality is more effective than telling a story. Listed below are the approximate calorie counts from some of your favorite foods. The first six are from Michael F. Jackson, Ph.D. (no, not **that** Michael Jackson!) executive director of the Center for Science in the Public Interest. The remainder of the foods are from several different sources, but equally of the "eye opening" caliber. **Warning! Do not feel guilty after reading these. Guilt may be hazardous to your health.**

Here are the findings based on normal serving sizes:

Cheese fries with ranch dressing	3,010	calories
Chinese orange beef	1,770	"
Large movie popcorn w/ butter	1,640	"
Kung Pao chicken	1,620	"
Carrot cake from a famous restaurant	1,560	"
Fettuccine Alfredo	1,500	"
B.K.'s: orig. double Whopper w/cheese value meal	1,980	"
Hardee's: Monster Burger	1,060	"
Domino's: Meatzza feast, 3 slices	1,130	"
Jack in the Box: Bacon Ult. Cheeseburger	1,120	"
Subway: 12 inch Meatball Classic Sub	1,054	"
Taco Bell: Mucho Grande Nachos	1,320	"

Most of these are an entire week's worth of calories for many African countries! Looking at these makes it easy to understand why America is bulging at the seams in more ways than one!

"What, me worry?" –Alfred E. Newman
(Maybe he wasn't talking about his belly,
but it makes you wonder.)

Being taken off the list of being classified as obese is extremely important in your fight for longevity. Yet, by itself, it is not one of the ten steps to longevity and better health because taking off the weight involves many different steps, not just a simple decree to action. By following this program, though, your weight will fall off naturally. Or you could just purchase one of those stupid electrical devices that you connect to your midsection and observe it "just melt the inches off" while *you* are watching *Everybody Loves Raymond!* Unfortunately you'll have spent a small fortune on batteries and you will be long gone before you'll lose any weight with that gimmick.

Chapter 3:

Who's in Charge?

Who's actually in control of your health and well-being? Most people would have to say that their doctor is the one pulling the strings when it comes to charting a course for their health. What's the first thing you do every time you get sick? You probably pick up the phone and try to get in to see your already over-booked M.D. Unless it's an emergency, your appointment will be three weeks from next Thursday. By then, you're either better or totally exhausted from fighting whatever it is that you may have caught. So you go to his office, sit in the waiting room for two hours when the assistant finally calls your name. "Thank God," you think, "that *Popular Mechanic's* magazine was getting pretty boring." Now, after being led to your little cubicle (by the way, every sick and contagious patient that your doctor has seen in the last millennium was in that tiny room leaving behind plenty of germs to share with you!), his assistant takes your pulse to make sure you're alive, strangles your arm reading your blood pressure, and asks you all sorts of important diagnostic questions like, "Do you have insurance to pay for this visit?" If she gets a "yes" answer, she then leaves. Another twenty minutes go by. Then, the drums roll, the curtains are pulled back and your almighty doctor, the miracle worker rushes in the room. Three minutes later, with prescription in hand, you spend another twenty minutes paying and then blocking out another half day, three weeks from now to see him again.

It's not that your doctor doesn't care about you and your health. He just doesn't have the time, nor does he wish to be put into the position of being your one and only *Almighty Healer.* He has got to run too many patients through those doors on a daily basis because of his ever-expanding overhead. There is malpractice insurance, expensive equipment, salaried personnel, rent, private schools for his children and the country club membership. He doesn't have the time to see how you are doing in your life or discover that your spouse left you, your career has been derailed, your mortgage is in arrears and your dog just died. That you also have been to see another doctor for a completely different problem who prescribed you a different medicine that may interact with what he just prescribed, and that a palm-reader told you that, "your time in this world is up." Your M.D. doesn't know this, but **if he took the time to find out more about your present environment, his diagnosis may be a little different.** He may have actually wanted to prescribe an entirely different drug more useless that the one he just did.

On dangerous grounds

As important as your doctor should be in the management of your health, did you know that it's downright dangerous to visit him? Over 7,000 deaths annually are caused by prescription errors alone! That doesn't even include misdiagnoses. These were just mistakes in the filling of the prescription by either the doctor, the pharmacist or maybe as a result of the infamously horrible handwriting of doctors. These numbers, by themselves, would be enough to recall any other product or service sold on America's store shelves!

Let's again ask the question concerning to whom you want to entrust your health. Again, most of us would put our trust in our modern and wonderful health-care system to guard and protect them for the rest of their lives. **Wrong answer!** In fact, way wrong. **The American health-care system doesn't give a damn about you and will do everything in its power to deny you coverage, over-charge you and in general, make your life miserable.** Do you sometimes feel privileged to even have health coverage? Ever had to actually be admitted into a hospital? Unless you're just visiting your Aunt Louise, the experience probably demoralized you, caused you to lose faith in your fellow man, gave you heartburn and sent you into a depression . . . and that was before you got past the admitting desk! Our hospitals are under-staffed, under-trained, many times obsolete and over-worked. **You need to do your absolute best to stay out of any and all hospitals whenever possible.** Why? Because being admitted into a hospital can be outright bad for your health, as in dangerous or even lethal!

An Illinois study found that the average hospital makes 40 drug errors a day! In the 36 hospitals they examined, one in five attempts to give the medicine needed was done in error. One in five medications, which comes out to one of every two patients given meds were affected . . . you shouldn't like those percentages.

A Dr. Gerald Barnes saw thousands of patients at several medical facilities for over 20 years. He treated people for everything that a general practitioner should from colds to heart disease. It's too bad that he wasn't even a licensed doctor! It didn't matter that he was arrested 5 times and spent 2 years in prison for related convictions. He went right back to practicing medicine without a license. Why didn't any of the medical facilities that he worked at bother to check his credentials? Were you one of the patients he treated? He may have been pretty good, maybe even proficient, but do you care to take that kind of gamble with your life? Worse, do you care that our health-care system is so broken that Gerald Barnes was able to pull off this charade? How many Gerald Barnes' are there in this country?

We're not through in the hospital, yet. You've already heard of the amputations done on the wrong limbs, which may sound funny now, but probably wasn't very funny to the patient. You may have also heard of the two neurosurgeons, one who had to go to the bank and another one that took his lunch break, neither activity was considered out of the ordinary except that their patient's skulls were still in multiple pieces when they left the operating room to take care of their personal chores! How many other types of compromising events happen in our surgery rooms on a daily basis that are covered up by their staff? Are they just leaving instruments sewn up inside of your chest cavity, or are there other worse occurrences? This next story was in the newspaper recently. Two children with cancer received chemotherapy overdoses in one Baltimore hospital. One child went deaf, the other eventually recovered. It seems that their hospital staff doubled up on the medication they were supposed to receive. Oops!

A sixteen-year-old Mexican girl lost her life recently. Seems the heart and lungs used in her multiple organ transplant were the wrong blood type . . . oops again! You would think that the blood types would be the first thing that they would check, but each party involved assumed that the other checked for that *minor* detail.

There have also been several stories in the last couple of years about hospital personnel, usually nurses, who seem to get a thrill out of watching someone die. One such nurse in Texas is suspected of "aiding" in the death of over 20 older patients. Unfortunately, these types of cases are hard to prove (possibly because the only witness to the crime is no longer around), so we will probably only see more of these cases in the future. The majority of those patients were probably going to die anyway, but the guilty hospital personnel decided to play God. How nice of them. Hello, Dr. Kevorkian! It seems that you now have some competition!

A University of Pennsylvania study precipitated by the concerns about our nationwide shortage and resulting over-working of nurses, found that the number of patients a nurse cares for *can* directly affect whether a patient lives or dies. Researchers found that patients had a greater chance of an early funeral after surgery when their nurses had more patients to care for. This study released in the *Journal of the American Medical Association* showed that a heavy workload not only caused job burnout and unhappiness, but also a 7% increase in death within 30 days of surgery for these unlucky people. Unfortunately, this gruesome statistic makes sense. So you better hope your nurse doesn't have too many patients, but has plenty of patience.

Shouldn't your nurse's work load be the last thing that you should have to worry about while laid up in a hospital after major surgery?

If you are lucky enough to survive all the personnel who have no business working in a hospital, and if you happen to receive the correct drugs while you are under their care, **all you have to do now is to survive all of the many parasites, viruses and bacteria that are unique to, and are thriving very well inside of hospitals only waiting for you to arrive. The American hospital can kill in ways not intended to, proven by the fact that over 100,000 patients a year die from infections and ailments they received while in a hospital.** As an example, you enter a hospital to get your tonsils out, contract a very nice antibiotic-resistant bacteria (there are several to choose from), and then die before leaving this tremendously less-than-sterile establishment. Did you ever wonder why they have you fill out all of the financial paperwork *before* you step foot inside your less-than-private room? Not many businesses make you pay prior to having services performed.

There are many, many antibiotic-resistant bacteria thriving very comfortably in most hospitals making your number 1 goal to stay away from them whenever possible. By the way, these resistant bacteria are considered to be of epidemic proportions by the Center for Disease Control (CDC). More on that later.

A hospital should be one of your last options in taking care of your health. Don't just refuse to go because of what you have read, but by practicing preventive care you can keep yourself away from them as much as possibly. By minimizing your hospital stays, you'll increase the chance of surviving a little longer and spend a whole lot less money along the way. Remember, this game of life is all about percentages, and you want the numbers in your favor as much as is possible.

The results of the following studies and findings illustrate several more examples of why not to trust anyone other than yourself to protect your future health. Government researchers found that a type of knee surgery done more than 300,000 times annually to ease arthritis pain (osteoarthritis) is "worthless and perhaps even harmful." A large group of older Americans who had arthritic knees were sliced open; some were worked on, the others just sewn back up. The ones with only the incisions were up quicker and found better relief than the group that actually got their money's worth! (We will also talk about the power of your mind later on. This is one extreme example of mind over matter.) That particular type of surgery was, and is, considered a waste.

Lotronex, a drug used to treat Irritable Bowel Syndrome, usually in women, was pulled off the shelves after being linked to a number of hospitalizations and deaths. This drug was on the market for six months before being yanked. The makers of Coumadin, a popular blood thinner, are involved in a class action suit claiming "false and misleading" advertising. What exactly were they misleading us on? The acne drug isotretinion (Acutane) has been linked to depression in several hundred people since its inception. More than 100 were hospitalized (bad move in itself!) and 41 committed suicide. (One was the kid who flew a plane into a Florida Federal Office Building shortly after 9/11/01.) At least they died with a clear face! Such a nice drug!

A recently released study showed that more than 10% of newly marketed prescription drugs have serious side effects that do not show up until long after the drug debut. How does this happen when it takes so long to get a drug on the market? Wasn't there plenty of time to look for these side-effects? Doctors are being advised to allow these new drugs a few years of "seasoning" and to only prescribe older drugs that already have a proven track record of side effects and deaths. Yes, and with the overwhelming marketing done by pharmaceutical companies, I'm sure **that's** gonna happen real soon . . . when pigs fly.

Have you been prescribed heartburn medication recently? Taking too many can increase your risk of developing an ulcer. Did your doctor recommend any dietary changes first? Probably not. Your stomach produces acids (hydrochloric acid, for one) for a reason. Stopping their production is not usually a good idea, nor does it solve the original problem.

There are hundreds and hundred of other examples, but hopefully you get the picture. We are the most advanced country on the face of the earth and many wonderful inventions and discoveries happen every day, but sometimes traditional and time-proven practices are better than newer shortcuts and compromises. Maybe your grandmother really did know best!

Doctors are human, just like the rest of us. They get tired, cranky, are overworked and make mistakes. Do you want to be the recipient of an error by your doctor, either in diagnosis or treatment of any problem? Take a look at the men of the cloth. If they can make as many mistakes as we have found out about, then surely your favorite doctor can be susceptible to errors. What's more, just as with what has happened in the Catholic Church and in publicly traded corporate management, doctors too, are not accountable for their actions. Either there is no regulation in place or they are in charge of it themselves. As an example, the Texas State Board of Medical Examiners, the agency (of fellow doctors) that has pledged to protect the citizens of Texas, has shown over and over again that it does not. The agency has routinely forgiven surgeons, many times more than once, who have botched operations. It overlooked physicians who misdiagnosed cancers, maimed infants and caused unnecessary sterilization of women. **In fact, from 1997 to 2002 it revoked *no* licenses of any doctors for committing *any* errors!** I guess all the Texas doctors are perfect. The agency has failed to investigate any of the one thousand annual claims of misconduct it receives. Oh, they have pulled licenses . . . for drug convictions, for practicing medicine while a licenses was suspended, for mail fraud, sexual misconduct, inappropriate prescriptions (diet pill doctors come to mind), and alcohol abuse. No, this wasn't a list of former priests; these were your doctors! Where is their motivation to fly straight when they are not held accountable for their own actions? What will cause them to be responsible for the mistakes made in their chosen profession? Obviously, most doctors are honorable, not unlike the general population of our country, but how do you know that yours is beyond reproach? I'm sure that you will not settle for anything less that the best when it comes to your health, but the system in place now does not give you the protection that you need nor is it easy for you to do the necessary research.

Take all of the problems mentioned above with the fact that over 40 million Americans are without health insurance today, and the ones that do spend too much time fighting for the coverage they deserve. Add that to the reality that we as a nation are not geared toward preventative care, and you will find the following statistic, mentioned previously, even more interesting: **The World Health Organization ranked the U.S. overall health-**

care quality 37th best in the world! What??? How could 36 countries be ahead of us? Aren't we the best at everything? Apparently not. France and Italy were judged the best and a whole lot of "Mickey Mouse" countries were judged better than us. There is no excuse for that, but unfortunately it's what we have to live with. The National Academy of Sciences recently released a report stating that the United States health-care system is in crisis and in need of immediate attention. According to their administration, *"The health-care delivery system is incapable of meeting the present, let alone the future needs of the American public. The cost of private health insurance is increasing at an annual rate in excess of 12 percent, much higher than the rate of inflation. Individuals are paying more out of pocket and receiving fewer benefits and one in seven Americans are uninsured while that number is on the rise."* They also mentioned the 100,000 people dying from medical errors each year. **Although we as a nation can fix this problem . . . eventually, it should be obvious that it would be much easier to fix ourselves individually by practicing preventative care, and then just keep ourselves out of the path of this broken-down, out-of-control monster.** Care for an HMO on the rocks?

We, as a society, put way too much emphasis on the gods of western medical science. What's wrong with that philosophy besides all of the dangers mentioned above? Plenty. First of all, they really have limited training. They are schooled very well in anatomy, biology, chemistry and have a vast knowledge in being able to recognize disease and structural problems. Please, don't get me wrong, if you break a bone, are in a car wreck or find an abnormal cantaloupe-sized tumor growing on the side of your head, you need to visit a doctor. You also need to see one for your annual check-ups. The medical community's strong point is in analysis and diagnosis. They can set bones, remove growths, tell you if you have a disease or a herniated discs. **One of the crucial areas that the medical profession is lacking in, however, is in**

preventive care. Most any time that you see doctor for an ailment, he is going to prescribe a drug and tell you to take it easy for a couple of weeks. That's fine, except all that your doctor has done was to give you a Band-Aid! **Whatever he prescribed may have gotten rid of the immediate problem you had, but did nothing to discover why it happened in the first place or to take steps to keep it from happening again. The medical profession does not do a good job of recognizing the relationship between the different functions of your body and how they relate to your overall health. They work in a strictly reactionary mode using pharmaceuticals as their primary means of treatment.**

Proper exercise, as an example, has the ability to ease emotional stress that may cause depression by creating a brain chemical neurotransmitter called serotonin. This chemical creates a calm feeling plus it allows you to sleep better. When's the last time your shrink or doctor prescribed exercise? When's the last time he ordered you to begin an exercise program because if you didn't you won't make it another ten years? I didn't think so. Exercise should be a crucial part of your preventative care, but you're not going to hear that from your doctor. He's not going to tell you to eat better and supplement your diet with antioxidant-type substances even though those two things may keep you out of his office. Don't misunderstand my point of view. Doctors should play a very important role in your overall health-care program, but they don't want the burden of being considered your only option. Besides, I'm sure most would prefer a little lighter workload and a happier, healthier clientele.

The whole purpose of preventative care is to keep you healthy, keep you out of the doctor's office, give you the energy you require and prolong your life as long as you can. Best of all, it puts *you* in control. **If given the chance, your body will heal and mend itself. It will create its own natural enzymes, vitamins and chemicals to bring about the balance it needs to stay healthy.**

Plus, if there is a lack of anything, it will use minerals, vitamins and proteins that you feed it to supplement what it already possesses, in its fight to keep you healthy.

Things happen in your body for a reason. You don't just get a cold or the flu for no apparent reason. Arthritis doesn't just show up on your doorsteps unannounced and, God forbid, cancer doesn't gain a foothold in your system without some weakness somewhere in your immune system. Why hasn't your doctor explored any of these avenues? One of the answers is that he doesn't have the training in this area. Doctors are not schooled in nor do they usually have an interest in preventative care. They are taught how to recognize disease and what to prescribe to bombard it out of your body. To hell with the side effects! An M.D. is to your body what your mechanic is to your car. If it's broke, take it in to the shop and he will fix it. They have the tools, the training and the know-how to fix what you can't. You know not to give your car an inferior grade of gasoline. You don't need your mechanic to tell you that. If your tires are worn, you can see it for yourself. When it's dirty, you wash it and when it's time to change the oil, you do . . . sometimes. Your mechanic has a very specific role in the health of your vehicle and your job is to stay away from him. The same goes with your doctor. The better you treat your body, the less you'll see of him. That should be by design.

Now is the time for your solo

It should be obvious that your doctor is not the one best suited to be in control of your health. Neither are your family and friends. **The only one that knows your body best, has the most to gain, and is the only one that really cares what happens to it is . . . you. You are the one in control of your future health, no one else.** Why is it that you'll blindly follow what your three-minute doctor tells you, but you won't hesitate to get another opinion from a different auto mechanic? **You tend to take better care of your car than you do your health.** Your doctor doesn't have time, is not up to date on all of the recent studies and findings (also because of a lack of time), is not accountable by his profession and many times is swayed by the salesmanship of his local pharmaceutical representative. Your family and friends want the best for you, but don't usually have the intestinal fortitude to tell you what you **need** to hear instead of what you **want** to hear. Since most disease is preventable, why haven't they told you to stop smoking, quit eating so damn much of the wrong foods, abstain from alcohol, and get your lazy butt out of your Barcalounger long enough to exercise? Most of us really need occasional "tough love" from family and friends, but seldom ever get it. It's easier to be your buddy than your mother. So that is why your long-term health is up to you and no one else. Someone has to drive and it looks like you'll be the one.

What you will find in this book are most of the tools that you'll need to regain your youthfulness; and much of the energy and vigor you need. It may take a gargantuan effort by some, and at least a degree of discipline by others, but everything that you will need is outlined in these ten steps. Follow these guidelines and your body will thank you many times over.

Chapter 4:

Does Modern Medicine Have the Answer?

As you read in the previous chapter, you know that the response to this question is pointing toward no. Actually, more like a resounding no! However, from Western medicine's point of view, the response is, "Yes, we do have the answer." However, their solution to improving your health is always the same. The fix offered by researchers, scientists, and the remainder of the Western medical community is, "Let's find a drug to treat any problem that you may have." (Ask yourself if they have ever offered anything else? After all, you can't patent and make much money from something that is readily available on this earth.)

Western medicine has moved, or more aptly has been shoved, to a reactionary mode. The wonder drugs of the '50s seemed to usher in a new era in medicine by leaning toward a pharmaceutical-based answer to America's health problems. For every problem, companies were discovering a patentable cure either by mimicking something found in nature, like aspirin, to the array of synthetic drugs offered today. As the American investor continues to push for short-term profits, the pressure is on for pharmaceutical companies to perform; and perform, they have! Drug companies are very profitable. Last year, the five most profitable drugs alone had combined sales of well over $14.5 billion. There is absolutely nothing wrong with corporate profitability, since, after all, that is the American way.

What is suspect, though, is the method of operation used by pharmaceutical companies. By following doctors all the way from med school to internship and finally to their place of practice, they have managed to convince the medical profession to use their particular product. From sponsoring many of the supposedly unbiased research studies to underwriting medical schools and finally deluging doctors with promotional information and tons of samples, drug companies have firmly implanted themselves within the medical profession, moving us further and further away from the world of preventative care.

Blame isn't entirely on the doorstep of the drug company marketing department. After all, doctors receive minimal, if any, training in preventative care and most don't share the belief that *if given the chance, your body will heal itself.* They have been swamped with problem after problem and frankly don't have the time to think about any of the other choices that preventative care has to offer. They are too busy putting out the proverbial fires and aren't spending enough time educating their patients in the virtues of taking proper care of themselves. **The entire medical community, including the organizations formed to regulate them, are not in the business to promote health. Rather, they are geared toward *managing disease,* not preventing it. Because of that, they will always be reacting to problems and not preventing them.**

A consumer advocacy group called *Public Citizen* is trying to get a drug used to fight the affects of rheumatoid arthritis banned, citing reports of liver failure and cancer in a number of Americans using this drug. The FDA's answer? Analysis shows that it is no more dangerous than *other* competing drugs. Isn't that reassuring!

Preventive care should always be your first step in guarding your health. Again, the emphasis is on **you** and **your** control over **yourself.** Stop disease and unwanted germs from either entering your body or massacre them before they gain a foothold inside of your system. Maybe the established world of Western medicine just assumes that you will not, or that you are incapable of taking care of yourself. Unfortunately, they have a strong case. As a society, we generally don't want to take the time or make the effort to build our body's defenses enough to create good health and avoid having to deal with doctors, drugs and disabilities. Oh, we can talk a good game, but when it comes down to actually taking the necessary action, many times the easier path is traversed. Now is the time for you to correct that philosophy and give yourself all the tools necessary to improve your health and extend your time above ground.

More and more articles are published each day showing that mainstream medicine is oriented solely toward medicating you. **Yes, they want to heal you, fix whatever the problem is, and in their own way improve your health, but the only way they know is through drugs . . . side-effect causing drugs, given *after* you become ill.** Think about these examples and the messages they project.

Parade Magazine printed an article written by Dr. Isadore Rosenfeld on rheumatoid arthritis in April of 2002. It was a thorough article on the analysis and treatment of this crippling disease, until Dr. Rosenfeld made the following statement when talking about DMARDs, a certain type of medicine recently developed to help fight the disorder. *"DMARD's can cause anemia and reduce the number of white blood cells and platelets, leaving you vulnerable to bleeding. They also can damage the liver, lungs and other organs. However, this potential toxicity should not deter you from trying them, as long as you are monitored carefully by your doctor."* What??? Do you want to take any drug with those possible side effects? It sure is easy for your doctor to "monitor" you since *he* is not the one taking these potentially harmful drugs. Why don't you just swallow diazinon or some other poison while you're at it? Just let your doctor monitor you. Instead of these drugs, the recommendation should involve a change in diet, a loss of weight and an appropriate exercise program. Throw in some supplements geared toward healing your joints and now you have a good, comprehensive program that may take a little longer but will prove to be a lot less dangerous and much better for you in the long run. After you have tried all of the above for a long enough period of time and you still suffer from rheumatoid arthritis, then, and only then, should you try the medication. (More than likely, you'll have cured the problem and won't need the medication.)

In another health magazine talking about fitness, the writer stated, "Researchers in Scotland are developing a class of drugs capable of fooling your body into thinking it's exercising, even though your [fat ass] is watching TV." (I threw in the "fat ass" part.) The drug is supposed to increase your metabolism and reduce your risk for diabetes while it helps you lose weight. Gee, I thought exercise accomplished the same thing. Why try and invent a solution for a problem that is sure to have side effects (they all do), when the solution is already there? Fitness in a bottle? Remember, if it sounds too good to be true, it usually is.

There have been several studies recently demonstrating that decreasing your overall caloric intake each and every day will improve your chances for living longer. This is actually good research and is really the only proven way to extend your life. We'll discuss this program later, but an article on it demonstrated the same, "let's drug them" mentality shown by our medical gods. In it the author stated, "It increases the likelihood that we will find pharmaceuticals that will mimic (increasing your metabolism) this effect." Again, eating less food is the proper solution, but go ahead and stuff yourself until you are sick. We have a pill that will work it off for you. Bring this drug out into the world and you will never see a more misused prescription ever. It will fly off the shelves . . . time to buy stock in that company! Never mind the consequences for taking the drug instead of changing your lifestyle. By the way, it's unlikely that it will ever work. Overeating has way too many harmful effects to be countered by some pill.

There are countless other examples of how America has been brainwashed into believing that the only source of relief from disease and suffering is through synthetic, side-effect-causing drugs, but we will move on.

In the previous section, several examples were mentioned of botched surgeries, mistakes made by tired, overworked hospital staff, criminal acts by medical personnel and lovely little antibiotic-resistant bacteria waiting to kill you while you visit your favorite hospital. In fact, the distinguished *New England Journal of Medicine* published a study recently entitled, "Risk Factors for Retained Instruments and Sponges after Surgery"! Losing medical instruments and supplies *inside* of the bodies of surgical patients is so common that it warranted doing a study on it?! (By the way, the study concluded that because of the excess recesses, obese patients tended to keep more of the hospital supplies inside of them than skinny folks . . . another reason to lose weight! And no, I didn't make that up.)

Ladies, here's one for you. Ever had gynecological surgery? For decades, medical students have been allowed to exam your pelvic area after you were anesthetized (asleep), without your permission! In other words, you enter the operating room, get knocked out, and then a hoard of wet-behind-the-ears medical students are invited to come inspect your private areas. Nice, huh? Did this happen to you? If you had the procedure done in a medical school, like the Harvard Medical School, chances are that until the late '90s this could have happened to you. By the way, many times it was the students raising complaints that brought about the change. Now, the consent forms that you sign allow them to do this. You may want to read these more carefully.

The bottom line is this. Not only is the one-sided reactive solution of drugging the American public not the answer to our health woes, the overall lack of care and respect when it comes to dealing with your body makes it a dangerous proposition to put your future entirely in the hands of the Gods of Western Reactionary Medicine. You need to grab control of your health and start steering it toward smoother roads by practicing preventative care and staying away from all those potholes.

Part 2:

10 Steps to a Long and Healthy Life

Step 1:

What's the Score?

It's a lazy weekend afternoon, you turn on the tube and there is a football game that holds some mild interest to you. What's the first thing you would like to know besides who hid the remote? You want to know what the score is and who is winning, right? The same holds true if you are personally attending a game, whether it involves one of your kids, grandkids or your favorite professional team. The game has already begun when you arrive and you need to find the present status of the contest. The same could be said for a lecture you walk into, a play, a sitcom, an auto race, etc. You need to assess the situation and perhaps find a point of comparison.

Well, before you can embark on *any* journey designed to improve your health, one that is going to allow you to live longer, you must first find out where you stand at the present time. What kind of health are you in now? Not ten years ago, not ten months prior. Now. So, what kind of shape are you presently in? We're not talking about just how you look. Anybody can look great for their age, but how is your cardiovascular health? Do you have any type of major ailment that you are aware of? The big caveat is "that you are aware of." **Fact: As you age, your susceptibility to crippling ailments increases significantly, some you may already have and not know about.** Approximately 300,000 Americans are HIV positive and don't know it. There are approximately ten million borderline diabetics in America that don't even realize they are about to become the unlucky recipient of this crippling disorder, and those numbers are sure to increase as we baby boomers age. Could you be one of them? You are at a greater risk of contracting diabetes, especially if you are inactive and overweight. Do you have any colon polyps? One hundred percent of all colon cancers begin as polyps, which are undetectable other than by specific testing. **The older you get, the greater chance you have of contracting cancers of many types, suffering from vascular, digestive, or even emotional problems, all of which can shorten your life significantly.**

It is extremely important to have a starting point in your quest for good health and longevity of life. One reason is to gauge how well you are doing and to at least sub-consciously gauge your progress. Positive feedback can't hurt. Sometimes you need that extra boost to keep you motivated when things may not seem to be going your way, and we all know that happens from time to time in any endeavor you undertake. This program is all about progress, but you will invariably hit some plateaus along the way and seeing how far you have come may help lift you out of the doldrums. Whether it's blood pressure, cholesterol level, weight, body-fat percentage or even the time that you are able to now ride a bike or run a treadmill, knowing how far you have come can help tremendously. You'll be on cloud nine when you discover that your cholesterol dropped 30 points!

Besides determining what ailments and life shortening markers you have now, you may be able to determine your propensity toward future problems too. That may be even more important than fixing your present predicament. If you can see an ailment heading your way, you have a lot better chance at stopping it cold in its tracks. In other words, if your serum-cholesterol and blood pressure is rather high and your father died fairly young from a heart attack, then guess what? Mr. "The Big One" is probably planning on visiting you long before he is invited. So tailor your program *especially* to reduce those two markers, lose some weight, eat better, and exercise and maybe he'll find a more receptive player, like the idiot at work that won't retire from the position you have deserved for the last eight years!

No one knows how long you are going to live. Not me, not you and certainly not your doctor; but the more that you can do now, while you are still relatively young and/or in good health will go a long way in lengthening your life. With the advances in medical science today, chances are that you will live longer than your parents did, but not necessarily to the degree of comfort you might like. All the more incentive to gauge where you are now and be better prepared for what lies ahead. The great Mickey Mantle, before his death said, "If I knew that I was going to live this long, I would have taken better care of myself." That wouldn't have taken much. . . The Mick knew how to live it up as well as anybody. An Oklahoma country boy was the toast of the town in the Big Apple. He was a god to normally sane, high-powered corporate CEOs whom, among other things, would never allow him to buy his own drink. The Mick probably never bought one from the day he landed at Yankee Stadium till the day he died. He had a great time. Unfortunately his liver and the rest of his vital organs didn't. The liver transplant he received was too late.

Mick's father and many other male members of his family died of heart disease very young and poor Mick assumed that he would too. Most of them didn't make it out of their forties, which wasn't so unusual in the years after World War II. The life expectancy of the average American went from fifty in 1920 to well over eighty today, so although it wasn't that much of a stretch for Mick to make that assumption after the fact, it was probably more of a subconscious observation. More than likely, it was merely a "hind sight" look at his life after it was too late. Can you imagine how good he *could* have been?

But his observation brings us to one of the two major steps that you need to take in the beginning stage of this program before moving on to the real meat of this plan. Mickey Mantle knew how his past relatives met their demise and you should, too. Get the family tree out. You need to investigate how your parents, uncles, aunts and grandparents died and what other ailments that they may have suffered leading up to their deaths. Did they die rather young? If they met their maker too early for their generation, what circumstances may have helped cause their last breath? If your uncle died of a heart attack, for instance, were there unusual family pressures that may have caused an abnormal amount of stress, adding unnecessary strain on his system that may have aided the heart disease? You need to find out how old they were and what kind of general shape that they were in at their death. Did they have any disease that wasn't mentioned as a cause of death, but certainly contributed to their demise, like diabetes? Did they smoke? Were they too heavy? Did they lead an active life? Were they known to knock down a few drinks . . . on too regular of a basis? Or were they just alcoholics? It's okay, in fact imperative to ask these questions; it may help lengthen your life. Don't feel uncomfortable asking your Aunt Louise about her husband who happened to be your blood relative. Did he have what is now known as Alzheimer's? You need to know. Write it all down and make some sense of it. It shouldn't be that difficult to come to some conclusions. The hardest part, like any project, is the accumulation of data.

However, just because you have this information doesn't mean that you are going to die from cancer since several relatives did. **All that this stage does is recognize some markers for you to be aware of when planning the rest of your life, because you are**

going to be the one in control of your life, not destiny, not genetics, not fate or dumb luck and certainly not your past history. Just because your family may have a predisposition toward a particular disease doesn't mean that you are going to suffer or die from it as a result. All it gives you is a section of your total health profile to help you better plan your future.

Cellular mutation of one kind or another causes most of the ailments that you have to worry about. The corresponding breakdowns in people's immune systems are the cause of 90% of the diseases out in this world, not genetics.

Don't buy into the genetics opinions that dictate, if your father died of a heart attack, then you probably will too. That's a crock! If you're predisposed to heart disease, then; begin exercising, lose some weight, get your cholesterol down, lower your stress levels, eat cholesterol-lowering foods and enjoy your long life. Your critics will probably be long gone before you decide to check out. With the advances being made in medical research everyday, you are being given tons of information that will help you fight any of the obstacles that you may later face. So begin today using what's called a **medical family tree,** a chart or graph if you like, or any other method that works for you and map out your family's medical history. Sources of information for this research include any living relatives, death certificates, hospitals, the military and insurance records. (You may need to prove your relationship to the deceased to obtain the data.) After compiling, look for any patterns and keep those in mind when charting your future health and well being. Make sure that you take this history with you when you visit your doctor, because that's your next step.

Dr./Mr. Goodwrench

When was the last time you went to see your doctor for a complete physical? That's what I thought. You probably treat your

Buick better than your body. If it needs a tune-up, an oil change, tires, battery or a transmission flush, then you're "Johnny on the spot." Get it washed, shine those tires, take it to the carwash weekly and protect it from its environment the best you can. Put a bra over the front end, keep it in the garage when you can, fly instead of drive that next vacation to keep the miles off your pride and joy. But if you are overly-fatigued, have frequent headaches or occasional chest pains, have gained an unusual amount of weight or just don't feel right, you just shrug it off to stress, age and your job.

How can you chart out the rest of your life if you don't have a clue where you stand right now? The obvious answer is that you cannot. In your teens, it was completely unnecessary. You gladly left the womb at or near twenty, and never looked back. Of course your doctor was the last person you went to visit and by the time you hit thirty, your family and their needs was more important than seeing some stupid doctor for your insignificant minor aches and pains. After all, that's just a part of aging, isn't it?

That's okay since we'll assume that you made it out of your thirties in fairly good shape and because of that you see no reason for getting a physical now. After all, "I'm bulletproof. Nothing can get me down." As Denzel Washington said in the movie *Training Day,* "King Kong ain't got nothing on me!" Of course his character died shortly after that, but that's beside the point.

Your teens, twenties and thirties were great years because your body's systems worked pretty darn well considering all the crap that you threw at it. All the junk food, drinks, pesticides and poisons, the "all-nighters," party here and party there and don't forget all the physical abuse you have endured. Your body worked pretty well and that's probably why you haven't gotten the physicals that you now need. Your body's hard work and phenomenal efficiency has been taken for granted, ignored and "dissed" day in and day out. Now, apologize to your poor body and pick up the phone.

You have to visit your family doctor for a complete physical. There is no way around this step. They are not God and shouldn't be treated with reverence, but for analysis purposes, they are "Mr. Goodwrench." If you have something wrong or some negative marker that you should keep an eye on, well, they will probably find it. Many health insurance companies make preventative care fairly inexpensive, so there shouldn't be any financial excuse. If you don't have insurance, and way too many of you don't, then shop around. There are plenty of providers that will give you a sizable discount if you do not carry insurance, and as a last resort, there are some home test kits that you can also use. (Please make home testing the absolute last place to have your health gauged since the obvious lack of objectivity and expertise could do more harm than good.)

You need to go through a battery of tests since most life-threatening illnesses can be averted if caught early enough. That should be obvious. In fact, you'll need to have some of these tests annually since many things in your beautiful body can change rather quickly. Your blood pressure can fluctuate overnight. A lump can appear in your breast in a matter of months. A number of things can cause your cholesterol to shoot up in as little as six months, and all sorts of hormonal imbalances, mineral deficiencies and cardiovascular problems can surface way too quickly to wait any longer than necessary.

Don't think that it can't happen to you, because it may already have. How many things have happened to and around you that you didn't think could? I didn't believe a psychology professor in college when he told us that one-third of us would have emotional problems in our lifetime. Actually, he was wrong . . . the figures are probably higher! You're not Superman or Wonder Woman (although it's okay for your spouse to believe that).

From the American Cancer Society, The American Heart Association and the National Osteoporosis Foundation, the following risks face the average woman over her estimated 80+ years on this planet:

The Average American Woman	Lifetime Risk
Osteoporosis related fractures	1 in 2
Heart disease	1 in 3
Skin cancer	1 in 5
Breast cancer	1 in 8
Lung cancer	1 in 17
Colon/rectal cancer	1 in 18
Uterine cancer	1 in 37
Ovarian cancer	1 in 59
Melanoma	1 in 82

I hate being considered average and I certainly don't like these averages. I assume that you don't either. Even the 1 in 82 chance of getting melanoma is too high, and that's why going to Mr. Goodwrench, better known as your family doctor, is critical to you having a long and healthy life. I would be willing to bet that the one person in three suffering from heart disease didn't take the precautions that you are about to, nor did they practice the healthy living habits that you are learning about here. No, they were just that stressed-out, over-weight, over-worked, fast-food junkie who lived next door. I hope he had a nice funeral.

So, what tests do you need and how often? That depends. Probably not the answer you were looking for though. While there are many routine tests that everyone needs, most patients seem to fall into one of two categories: those who get little or no routine examinations at any age, and those who have every little test that comes along whether they need it or not. Although you're better off erring on the side of too many tests and exams, they can be very costly and may cause more anxiety than necessary. Your personal check-up program, in order to be effective, needs to be tailored to your age, sex, specific personal circumstances and family history. Men don't need an annual prostate exam at 25 and women normally shouldn't need a mammogram at 20.

The following is a list of the most important tests needed, but, as far as frequency, consult with your physician.

Blood pressure

Blood pressure is simply the amount of pressure exerted upon the main arterial walls. It is highest when the ventricles are contracting (systolic) and lowest when they are relaxing and re-filling (diastolic). The two numbers generated when your B.P. is being measured refer to the systolic and diastolic pressure.

Most of the problems associated with blood pressure occur when the pressure is on the high side. Generally, if you have low blood pressure, you're going to know it by the amount of blood oozing from the knife or bullet wound that you just suffered, but low blood pressure can also be caused by internal bleeding.

High blood pressure, known as hypertension, wreaks havoc on your heart and arteries, and greatly increases your risk of heart attack and failure, stroke, kidney failure and a general overtaxing of all of your major organs. It also increases the possibility of Alzheimer's and other forms of mental decline. Put simply, having high blood pressure can kill you, sometimes instantly. It is not something to mess with.

The test for hypertension is quick, painless and should be done every time you walk into your doctor's office, even if you've only come in to pay your ever-expanding doctor's bill. A normal reading is 120 over 80. Anything up to 139 over 89 is considered slightly elevated and all numbers over that should sound the alarms.

The good thing about having an elevated blood pressure (if there are any positive things at all) is that it generally can be controlled by actions other than prescription medicine. In fact, avoiding blood pressure medicine is one of the easiest steps that you should take to rid yourself of unnecessary medicines since it can be accomplished through lifestyle changes like exercise, diet, supplements and stress reduction. Why bother with all of the potential side effects of drugs when you don't need to?

CHOLESTEROL

Cholesterol is the fat-like substance produced in the liver supplemented through foods that your body needs in order to function properly. **Without any cholesterol, you would die. Too much and you get the same results.** It's funny how life sometimes works. This waxy substance is the glue that holds your miniature cells together, the problem occurs when it builds up on the inside walls of your arteries, making it difficult for them to do their job while increasing the pressure on your heart and entire vascular system. The amount of your blood serum cholesterol is a general indicator of the condition of your arteries as it pertains to the efficiency of the flow of blood through your entire body . . . Just get it checked!

You have two different general types of cholesterol, one being good (HDL) and the other being bad (LDL). It's very simple. You want the HDL (good) to be 50 or greater and the LDL (bad) to be under 125 or so. The total cholesterol, although not as important as its component parts, should be less than 200.

Have your cholesterol tested now, if you haven't had it done recently, and repeat it at least every three to five years for the rest of your life. Again, having an elevated cholesterol count can lead to all sorts of cardiovascular diseases and is not something to take lightly. **As with hypertension, cholesterol is another problem that needs to be solved any way you can . . . without turning to pharmaceuticals.** A proper diet, exercise and supplement regime should take care of the problem. Yes, that isn't as easy as popping a few expensive pills ever day for the rest of your life, but beyond a doubt, the logical, natural way is much better. You will live a lot longer and be much healthier by avoiding the medicinal route. This is another example of taking control of your life and health and severing your dependence on others (like your doctor, pharmacist, and banker). You are the one in control, not Dr. Goodwrench! **By the way, the only way that you absorb cholesterol in your daily consumption of food is through animal products. Plant proteins and other plant foods contain no cholesterol.**

Blood work

For simplicity, we'll group most blood work into this category. Any complete exam is going to involve getting your arm poked and a few gallons of blood removed for review by several doctors, nurses, medical school students, technicians, insurance oversight committees, your Pastor, your next-door neighbor, J. Edgar Hoover and your bartender.

Your blood is a wonderful substance. There isn't a whole lot that can't be found out about your health by examining your blood. It's like looking at your diary. Today, Susan had some beef products, consumed over the legal limit of alcohol, had too much candy and was thinking bad thoughts about her boss. Maybe that's not the best analogy. How about the repair log your mechanic keeps on your car, assuming you use the same shop for most everything? You can get a reading on most of your major organs, test for diabetes and cholesterol, gauge your kidneys, test for cancers of many types and can check the condition of your prostate. All it takes is a few barrels of oil . . . no, blood. (You'll pay for it with the barrels of oil.)

Check your blood sugar level. If your glucose level is not

normal, it could signal diabetes. Elevated blood urea nitrogen (BUN) (no, I didn't make that up) can point to kidney disease. Have you checked your bilirubin count recently? I didn't think so. That should be done to verify that you haven't abused your liver too much. By the way, you do not want to lose the use of your liver. You need a healthy one to live, period. Everything that you put into your body goes through your liver, so remember that the next time you are contemplating that twelfth Jello-shot.

They need to check your PSA (prostate specific antigen), if you're a guy, to see if you're rear end needs to be violated. (You'll probably need one of those wonderful examinations every couple of years after reaching fifty.) Your white blood cells will be counted and if the total is over 12,000 per cubic millimeter, an infection may be visiting you. (This test explains the high cost of today's blood work. Someone has to work late counting each one of those little white blood cells. You sure hope that they don't lose count and have to start over.)

Is there too much uric acid in your blood? If so, you may have gout, which is a very painful form of arthritis. Let's not forget about your late-night escapades, so we better check for sexually transmitted diseases.

There is a new test that is a better indicator of heart disease than cholesterol levels and **looks for C-reactive proteins, or CRP in your blood.** This is a chemical that is necessary for fighting injury and infection with the latter being the important aspect here. **A ton of new evidence points to internal inflammation being the cause of many, many ailments, heart disease being one of them.** If you body has a high level of this protein, then it is fighting some internal inflammation that is doing it harm. This should be a red flag. It's interesting to note that a good diet and proper exercise lowers this protein tremendously by fighting the inflammation and/or injury that causes the protein buildup in the first place. **This is a new, but very important test and you will probably have to request that it be performed. Do not skip this one.**

Other tests

All women, and even men who have had bone fractures, should have their bone density checked beginning at age forty to keep their bones from becoming brittle. Osteoporosis is a huge problem with older women, putting many of them in wheelchairs long before needed.

Although a mammogram is not perfect, have one done annually after forty. Begin earlier if you have a family history of breast cancer. You're probably having pap smears done annually...good. There are 16,000 cases of cervical cancer each year in the U.S. and you don't want to be one of them. An annual PAP smear will reduce your chances of this cancer significantly.

Men, bend over and allow your doctor to "look up your address." (That's what my father called it.) At forty, begin having a prostate exam and at fifty, have your PSA checked (from your blood) every year for prostate problems. Keep your prostate healthy and "Woody" will stay around longer. Lose him and you'll lose your house when your wife leaves you for the twenty year-old pimply-faced pool cleaner!

Pair up cowboys and cowgirls. Both men and women should have the following tests done: Vision and glaucoma should be checked annually at age forty. You should have a full-blown colonoscopy done at fifty and if comes out negative, you're probably good for another five to ten years. This is not a fun test, but remember that **all** colon cancers begin as polyps, and they can be snipped while you are having the test done. By doing the complete colonoscopy, both the left and right sides of the colon are checked and that should cover 90+% of any polyps found. This is not a test to skip. **There is no more important test that you can take. By doing this, you may well eliminate colon cancers from your future. Don't take it . . . well, just take away half of that deck of cards. You are playing with fire.** By the way, this procedure's reputation is more severe than its reality. The worst part is not being able to eat the entire day before and then trying to choke down the required liquid that evening! After that and the Demerol, the procedure is easy.

Your hearing should be gauged every three years. At sixty-five, add a flu and pneumonia vaccine annually, increase the frequency of your eye exams to yearly also, and have your thyroid function checked. Get a tetanus shot every ten years for insurance purposes in case you step on that rusty nail or put one through your hand. You may want to talk with your doctor about the possibility of receiving any of the hepatitis series of vaccinations if you are at risk.

The chart on the following page should better summarize all the myriad of exams, poking and violations that you are going to have to endure, all in the name of good health. Hey, I'll bet your car doesn't like having his radiator flushed either, but he sucks it up, knowing that it will keep him running longer and that it will make you a happy camper. So, do the same for yourself and your family.

By the way, if you're having trouble getting quality time with your physician and it is frustrating you, try communicating with him or his staff by e-mail. As with the rest of our society, more and more doctors are keeping track of e-mails better than phone calls.

By exploring your family tree and allowing your doctor to explore your body on an annual basis, these two simple steps will go a long way in keeping you healthy for a long time to come. See you in the waiting room. I'll bring some good magazines!

Recommended Tests and Timetables

AGE	WHO	EXAM	FREQUENCY
Before 40	M/F	Complete physical	1–3 years
	F	Pap Smear	Annually (sorry)
	F	Mammogram	Annually, if at risk
	M/F	Cholesterol	1–3 years
	M/F	Blood Pressure	Annually
	M/F	Tetanus Booster	10 years
40–65	F	Mammogram	Annually
	M/F	Blood Work	Annually
	M/F	Cholesterol	1–3 years
	M/F	Blood Sugar	Annually
	M/F	Liver/Kidney Functions	3 years
	M/F	Prostate	Annually (sorry)
	M/F	Stool sample — colon	1–3 years
	M/F	Vision/Hearing	3 years
	M/F	Dental	Annually
	M/F	C-reactive proteins	Annually
50+	M/F	Bone Density	1–3 years
	M/F	Check skin for Cancer	Annually
	M/F	Full Colonoscopy	10 years
	M/F	Tetanus Booster	10 years
	M/F	Check pulse to see if living	annually
65+	M/F	Vision/Hearing/Dental	Annually
	M/F	Flu/Pneumonia Vaccine	Annually

Step 2:

Asleep at the Wheel

When's the last time you really got a good night's sleep? You woke up refreshed, bounced out of bed and were ready to take on anything and everything you encountered. That's what I thought. That may happen occasionally, but I'm willing to bet that it doesn't occur on a regular basis. Who cares? Quite simply, you should. This is, on one hand, the most obvious of all health problems that we face, but on the other hand **it's the most ignored and potentially dangerous issue that we, as a society, *don't* face.**

It's estimated that over half of our adult population doesn't get rejuvenating rest and the deep sleep needed on a regular basis. What difference does it make? All the difference in the world. Being overly tired has obvious problems, like falling asleep while driving along a two lane highway, having an accident and killing yourself and a busload of bingo-playing seniors. Okay, maybe that was a little extreme of an example. They were probably on their way to an outlet mall instead. How about missing appointments, not thinking clearly, not having the energy to do anything other than coming and going to work? Those are the obvious problems associated with sleep deprivation; but what's the real price we pay for staying up late to watch reruns of *The Beverly Hillbillies?* All the exercise in the world *and* a great diet will do you absolutely no good if your body doesn't rest sufficiently enough to rejuvenate itself. Even your car needs rest. It isn't designed to go 24/7 and neither are you.

By getting good restful sleep, your brain recharges, your body tears itself apart and then rebuilds itself at the cellular level. It's like an engine overhaul each and every night. Without it, your brain gets foggy and your body doesn't run on all eight cylinders. If you don't rest regularly, it's just a question of time before you start breaking down. **Lack of good and restful slumber affects the efficiency of every aspect of your body, including: your memory, energy level, blood pressure and, most importantly, your immune system.** It even affects your ability to lose weight by controlling the level of cortisol secreted, which, in part, controls your appetite and fat storage.

THE REAL COSTS OF SLEEP DEBT

We are sleeping an average of 20% less than our ancestors did just a century ago. That's about an hour and a half less every night! That amount of time can affect your *alertness* by up to 33%! A little less sleep than that can slow your *reaction time* by 10 to 15%! That's enough time to cause most accidents, whether they be at home or in your car. We have enough distractions around us already without having to worry about a slower reaction time!

With 40 to 50% of all Americans not getting the restorative rest they need, it is obvious that many of the accidents, problems and even catastrophes in our nation are at least partially a result of the effects of an overall lack of sleep.

Fact: Over 100,000 automobile accidents annually are directly caused by fatigued drivers.

Fact: Missing work because of sleep loss costs our country close to $50 billion annually in lost productivity, sick time and work related accidents.

Want more proof? Sleep problems were at least contributory factors in the following disasters:

1. The space shuttle Challenger exploded on January 28, 1986 killing its crew of seven. A presidential commission blamed the accident on the inattention of details by severely sleep-deprived personnel.
2. The Exxon Valdez accident happened because an exhausted crew-member took the helm after two days of heavy labor and not much sleep the previous night.
3. The Three Mile Island near meltdown in 1979 happened because the controlling worker had just changed to the night shift and had not adjusted to the regime. Inattention was blamed.
4. Chernobyl? Yes that, too.
5. Every year there is an 8% drop in traffic accidents the Monday following the turning back of our clocks one hour (allowing for an extra hour of sleep) due to the time change in late October. How many more lives could be saved?
6. Your team that lost the Super Bowl game did so because they were out too late the night before the big game. Somebody needs to pay for that one!

How many others went undetected? There are probably plenty more examples but that's not our immediate problem. We want to concentrate on fixing your sleep problems to help keep you from entering someone's trivia book. Yes, you probably have a problem with sleep. If you were well rested, you would awake every morning wondering why the world is moving so slowly while you whistled your way to work preparing to conquer the world.

The Red Badge of Courage

Overheard at the water cooler; employee number one: "Man, I'm bushed. I was up till 2:00 last night working on the Harris proposal and then had to get up at 6:00 AM as usual." Employee number two: "Ha! I went out with the guys from Dillon Enterprises, got home at 1:00 AM Stayed up until 2:30 before walking the dog. Up again at 5:45 AM!" Employee number three: "that's nothing. I haven't gotten a full-night's sleep since the Carter Administration" (Come to think of it, with the high interest rates and inflation associated with his administration, none of us did!) We seem to wear that sleepless zombie look like a badge of courage! The hero stands guard while the weak and timid sleep. What's up with that? Why do we punish our bodies over and over again and then boast about how our own particular insomnia affects our life?

The Benefits of Restful Sleep

The long list of benefits of getting a restful, restorative night's sleep includes: improving your immune system, repairing your muscles, bones, skin and other organs, lowering your blood pressure, giving you more energy to use during the day, increasing your overall brain functioning, quicker reaction time and allowing you the patience required to put up with more nagging from your in-laws.

Sleep is restocking time for your body. Hormones are circulated throughout your body, which assist in the repairing of all facets of your cells. Some of these are the growth hormones that are so abundant when you are young. After a period of time, your body stops making the excess amount of the hormone that allows you to grow, but still makes enough for the cellular repair process. However, something happened between then and now that not only has decreased the amounts of the hormones released, but also makes it more difficult for them to be circulated. That is one of the reasons that you don't recover from exercise as quickly as you used to, and are stiff and sore more than before. You need those hormones and restful sleep gives them to you.

Researchers have just begun finding the relationship between getting a good-night's sleep and your immune system. Technically your immune system consists of a complex array of several organs and cells including your bone marrow, lymph nodes, various lymphoid tissues of your tonsils, adenoids and appendix, your thymus located in the front of your chest and the Peyer's patches in your small intestines. They manufacture various antibodies called T and B cells that fight your never-ending (literally) battle against the things that want to do you harm, like disease, pollutants and telemarketers.

This all-important defense system needs the downtime to rebuild and recharge itself and to make its job of exterminating "unwanted aliens" a lot easier. All of the chemicals, enzymes and hormones that you need are created while you slumber. No rest, no properly performing immune system.

If beating Father Time is of any importance to you, then sleep is your Fountain of Youth. The reason for aging in the first place is the result of your cells being unable to rebuild themselves and not enough new cells being created to take their place. The time that this happens is while you are resting.

What really happens during sleep?

What really happens during sleep besides your kids sneaking out of the house and your car getting broken into? There are many different stages to sleep. The first stage involves a few minutes of drifting off, not yet sleeping. That's when you remember not feeding the dog for the last three days. So after taking care of that, you are back to the first drifting-off stage. Of course for the dog, it's a different story . . . he's thinking *"Man, my owner is worthless, can't even get anything to eat around here! I'm splitting the next chance I get...think I'll go over to his sister's house. She has a much bigger yard, and I hear you can eat right off her kitchen table! Yea, that's the ticket! I'll think I'll leave Ol' Worthless a little present on his carpet"* . . . Your dog never has trouble sleeping.

The second stage is characterized by your brain gearing down and can be characterized by a noticeable difference in brain waves as seen on one of those funny-looking EEG machines that measure brain activity. Stage 3 is the beginning of the deep sleep cycle and the 4th stage is the deep "delta" stage. The delta stage is extremely important. This is where your body rests and rebuilds itself. Most of the blood is actually diverted away from your brain and is circulated to the rest of your body, which by itself, should indicate that the increased blood flow is happening for a reason. Your temperature, breathing, and blood pressure drops, and hormones are secreted, especially growth hormones used mainly to repair and rebuild your muscle and other cells. Not much dreaming occurs during this stage because of an obvious lack of blood to your brain. This, by the way, is the stage that is most difficult from which to awake.

This semi-complete cycle last for about an hour to an hour and a half, then repeats itself with one difference: We didn't talk about the REM stage because it usually doesn't occur until the second cycle. REM stands for rapid eye movement and is at the light end of the sleep process. At this stage, about 25% of your total blood flow gets diverted **to** your brain and you begin dreaming or relearning your experiences of the day. The funny thing about this cycle is that part of your brain really doesn't know the difference between dreaming and actually being awake in relation to the thoughts and experiences you are having. The rapid eye movement is your mind actually following a dream. You're watching the dream as though it was really happening. However, directly before this cycle begins, an area of nerves deep within your brain stem relaxes your muscles, almost paralyzing them, probably so you don't make a fool of yourself thrashing around in bed acting out whatever you're dreaming. Note: researchers can actually turn off this mechanism and have done so in animals observing them acting out their dreams. Cheap thrills for laboratory nerds, I guess. Now if the researchers would do this experiment on humans . . . well, you can make up your own hilarious story to go along with the endless possibilities.

REM sleep occurs about every 90 minutes in adults and can last anywhere from 5 to 30 minutes in duration. However many hours you sleep will determine how many dreams that you will have. There is an interesting observation having to do with the EEG readings. The REM and the waves generated when you are awake are remarkably similar in their patterns (remember that the brain doesn't know the difference between the two). However the delta stage waves are completely different. The EEG readings are a direct result of positive and negative charges from the cells in your brain. When awake (or dreaming), the brain is completing hundreds of different functions at the same time, all competing with each other as they fire off charges, as shown on the EEG. The positive and negative charges end up canceling each other out and thus the small static readings. It's similar to a big evenly-matched battle where no one makes much progress. However, in the delta stage, the brain is supposed to be virtually inactive because of the lack of blood flow, but the EEG waves are very much in sync and have a distinctive ebb and flow as if they were rehearsing a finely choreographed dance. In this stage, while your *body* is "retooling" itself, your *brain* seems to be resetting itself. It could be that the REM stage tests all the different areas of the brain (doing a brain diagnostic) and the delta stage actually resets it. An interesting theory.

The bottom line is that you need both of these stages of sleep several times a night. Researchers have deprived people of each of these stages with the resulting energy loss, the slowing of reaction time, lack of quantitative reasoning and the inability to rebuild the immune system proving that the effects of sleep deprivation are not in your best interest!

So, how much good, uninterrupted sleep do you need? Good question. One in fact that only you can answer. Most experts seem to compromise on about seven to nine hours being the magical number, but that depends on how efficient your rest is and how many sleep cycles you can get in per night. **Any interruption in sleep disrupts these important stages and most all sleep problems are a result of interfering with those cycles several times a night for a variety of reasons. Stress, chronic pain, chemicals, snoring, and waking up maybe several times a night (not even remembering that you did) can all cause the sleep cycle to be short-circuited. Therein lies the problem. Lose the REM and Delta sleep stages and life becomes a struggle and challenge each and every day.**

GET RID OF THE OUTSIDE DISTRACTIONS FIRST

There are many sleep disorders that may be affecting you, but in order to explore the possibilities of purely medical problems we need to get rid of all the outside variables that may be contributing to your lack of good quality slumber. Chronic insomnia is nothing more than a general long-term lack of restorative sleep and not a specific disorder, so we'll refer to any sleep problems as insomnia. Your lousy sleep may be a result of simple environmental problems (specific to you) and not medical in nature. But as we have said, the end result of sleep deprivation can certainly turn into plenty of other medical problems besides just being tired!

There are several types of sleep-robbing life experiences. The inability to turn off stress will prohibit your brain from concentrating on the job at hand. Also, if you're in pain, especially in your joints, those "Houston, we have a problem" signals to the brain will halt your sleep. Fibromyalgia and arthritis problems, injuries, cramping, soreness and tightness in muscles, headaches, toothaches, tummy-aches, menstrual pains and an accidental right-cross punch from your spouse in the middle of the night can all cause your brain to short circuit the sleep process, making you a grouchy and tired person.

Do not underestimate these little nuisances' ability to keep you from sleeping soundly. You have to take steps to arrest any and all maladies that are affecting your precious slumber. Stretch or take a hot bath to relieve muscle stiffness and soreness. Take a pain-killer if nothing else works to get rid of a headache. Don't eat, especially spicy foods, before retiring. Exercise, but not directly before bedtime, to help fight the fibromyalgia and the arthritis symptoms. And of course, sleep far enough away from your spouse's jabs and punches!

Stress, the silent killer, that will be discussed in a later chapter, has the ability to keep you awake indefinitely. We all have several stress triggers, way too many to list, that have kept us up at night. There are, however, many things that you can do to alleviate staying up all night. If it's work related, keep it at work . . . in other words: finish your daily work at your office. Resolve what you can then and there, and make a list of things to do tomorrow before leaving today. If there is important work that you didn't get done, try to do it before you leave, if you can. If not, at least make a dent in it so you can feel a sense of accomplishment. If you work at home, keep sensible hours for work and try to use the same rules that you would if you worked in an office away from home. That is sometimes difficult to do depending upon your line of work, but make an effort regardless.

Note: Do not use your bedroom as an office. It is not conducive for sleep.

If you and your spouse are having problems, the bed can become a battlefield. That's not very conducive to sleep, either. (Boy, is that an understatement! Just beat the hell out of each other and get it over with.) Discuss disagreements several hours before going to bed so as not to be wound up upon retiring. Your body and mind need a cooling-down period before sleep. You can't very well run several miles and immediately expect to be able to fall directly asleep. Nor can you have too much excitement of any kind before sleep. Slow down, calm down and relax for at least an hour or so before bedtime for obvious reasons. Read a book or magazine. If you're still mad at your spouse and the problems haven't been resolved for some time, then you need to seek outside counseling. Yes, suck it up and get help. You won't be alone. Most of our society needs psychological help of one kind or another; it's not just you. A lack of sleep will do nothing positive for your problems and in fact will make them worse. **All** successful relationships are full of constant compromise. Now, if I can just get my wife to do all the compromising . . . Stress: know it's there and make a conscious effort to get it under control.

Exercising

Exercising (again not directly before bed) will release relaxing hormones (serotonin), will help you get rid of excessive energy, give you a sense of accomplishment and help alleviate the aches and pains associated with arthritis, chronic fatigue, fibromyalgia and just plain getting old. A long walk after dinner with your favorite loved one (quite possibly your dog, since he is the only one that understands you) is perfect. This will help the digestion process, work off some stress and get those hormones going.

Sleep aids

Several sleep aids are available whether they are over-the-counter or by prescription. Some of the prescription medications are: Benzodiazepines (Halcion, Restoril and Klonopin), Ambien, Trazodine, etc. You can purchase without a prescription: Nyquil, Sominex, Excedrin PM, Benadryl and a host of others.

Nutritional supplements include: melatonin, kava kava, St. John's wort (someone made a bad mistake in marketing when naming this herb!), valerian root, ginseng, Passion Flower (use this one just for the name!), and chamomile.

Stay clear of most of them. They may help you get to the point of sleep, but most of them will prohibit you from entering the REM or Delta stages that you need so badly. If, however, you are and/or have had horrible sleep habits (like not being able to get to bed at a regular time), then do whatever it takes to get into a routine. **Developing good sleeping habits is the first step in obtaining blissful and restful sleep.** The pills may be a necessity to get you there. However, discontinue them as soon as it is possible and certainly after a few days at the most. The exceptions to the list above involve valerian root and chamomile. These are fairly mild and have little side effects. The other supplements (not any of the drugs) have benefits in other areas such as depression, fatigue and mental functions and can be of use if sleep is not a huge problem.

SMOKING

If you smoke and also have a sleep problem, them this is another reason to quit. No, don't quit sleeping! We're talking about smoking . . . Nicotine is an addictive stimulant among its other wonderful traits and can keep you awake. Besides, if you smoke then you may have a smoker's cough, which can waken you also. Smoking is a nasty habit with no redeeming qualities and if it's interfering with your slumber, then stop anyway you can.

ALCOHOL

Alcohol also may relax you, but will certainly inhibit the deep stages of sleep that you need. A drink or two is probably okay, but you should limit it to early in the evening so it has a chance to get through your digestive system. Besides, you don't need another reason to get up in the middle of the night. Don't underestimate the power of liquor. *There are far too many Americans who have a drinking problem.* One or two drinks a night may not hurt, but any more than that can wreck havoc on your life and adversely affect the ones you love in many different ways. You don't have to be a slobbering drunk to have a problem. Most alcoholics handle the problem without anybody else knowing, which may be more dangerous than the drunks who are obvious. I'm not preaching for you to quit drinking. It can certainly have benefits, but like most anything else in life, moderation is the key. Give your life, liver and your immune system a break!

Top Ten Sleep Suggestions

If you will follow these ten simple rules outlined beginning on page 85, you should solve the vast majority of any sleep related problems. They are fairly simple, straightforward and can do more to improve your sleep than just about anything. They are the real "meat" of this chapter. **If you don't get enough good quality sleep on a regular basis, you *will* suffer. Whether it's a slower reaction time, dulled mental abilities or a compromised immune system, it will affect you. Since your system will not be regenerating, it will be slowly destroying itself.** You want that "Fountain of Youth?" Get the best quality sleep that you can and you'll successfully delay Father Time.

It's imperative that you make sure that you do not have any of the medical problems listed on the next page and in this section. If you do, then you must go to a doctor for advice, ASAP. The steps outlined here will help, but probably won't cure your medically-related sleep problems. One of our goals is to try and prevent any interruption of your sleep cycles during the night, but you may need medical assistance to achieve your much-deserved bliss.

Medical Problems

Do you suffer from sleep apnea or any of the other medical chronic insomnia problems? Here are just a few of them:

1. **Night-time eating syndrome.** This is self explanatory. Don't eat heavy or late in the evening. Don't go to bed hungry or full of food or liquids. Seek counselling if you cannot quit.
2. **Restless leg syndrome.** That's doing the Riverdance while sleeping. It's disruptive to your sleep cycles and will anger anyone sleeping with you. Stretching or taking a warm bath before bed may help.
3. **Conditioned Insomnia.** This is where you have become so stresses out because of not being able to fall asleep that you associate your bed with the anxiety it causes and thus it becomes a self-fulfilling prophecy.
4. **Arcadian Rhythms Disorder.** Your internal body clock is screwed up. We'll discuss the importance of regular bed times later.
5. **Sleep Apnea.** There are many different types of apnea, but in general it occurs when something actually stops you from breathing several (sometimes hundreds of) times a night. For this you should seek professional help. If you snore or gasp often, then this could be a problem that cannot be solved here. See a doctor. At least twenty million Americans suffer from sleep apnea alone. If you snore on a regular basis (don't worry, you'll know that you do because someone will have already told you this several hundred times!), then you have some sort of apnea. If you gasp while sleeping, then your throat is either obstructed or has collapsed and that is called Obstructive Sleep Apnea. Central sleep apnea is a neurological condition that causes your breathing process to stop or pause while asleep, thereby interrupting the sleep process.

Top Ten Sleep Suggestions

1. **A good mattress.** Are you still using that mattress that you hauled everywhere you lived during college? You know, the one that fell off the pickup truck twice on the way to the third floor loft above the taxidermy store. If so, it just may be time to say goodbye to it. I know the memories were . . . well we'll just say that they were memories. A good mattress probably isn't good for much more than ten years, if you're lucky. Judging by how many more aches and pains you probably have now as compared to your teens and early twenties, it's re-evaluation time for the bed. No one can tell you what kind of mattress you need, whether it's firm, soft, pillow-topped; whether it has springs, coils, down feathers, pecan shells, tortilla shells, shotgun shells, sea shells or whatever is the new craze. Make your own choice. A waterbed can be the greatest purchase you could make, or it can make you seasick. They now come with baffles, fiber-filled to different degrees of firmness, heaters and vibrators. There are air beds, adjustable beds, futons, etc. They all sound great! However the only way to know is to try different types, with your sleeping partner, if you have one. If you're thinking about having a mate, but you're not sure which person it will be, then take all of them bed shopping! Wouldn't that be lovely? If they all like a certain type of bedding, then you can't go wrong. Come to think of it, if your partner is not happy, then it doesn't matter if you're sleeping on clouds-you ain't gonna be happy. Bottom line: if your present sleeping vehicle is over ten years old or certain injuries now make it uncomfortable, then you need to reevaluate. Take your time; it's an expensive and long-term purchase.
2. **Snoozing environment.** Your bedroom needs to be cool, dark and quiet; kind of like a dingy bar without the smoke and obnoxious drunks. Studies show that the best sleep is obtained when your body temperature drops a little, so lower the thermostat and turn on the fan. You can also take a cool bath right

before bedtime to get your body temp started lowering. Also, light is the archenemy of sleep. Daylight, lamplight, bright TV light and a raging fire all wreck havoc on Mr. Sleep. It makes him very unhappy, and he returns the favor to you. Noise is also very distracting . . . what a brilliant statement that was. Like you're going to be able to sleep through gunfire, kids screaming, spouse yelling, TV blasting, neighbors partying and snoring. Make it quiet! Other than some white noise, which is background sounds like a fan, mini-waterfall thingies, low hum of a radio; do whatever works for you. Again, your bedroom needs to be cooler than normal, allow very little light in, and be as quiet as is possible. This is a big step towards a good night's sleep.

3. **Avoid stimulants.** Caffeine, tobacco, alcohol and meds need to be restricted severely. Stop all caffeine intake by mid-afternoon or you may be wired when you retire for the evening. If sleep is a problem, then you are just asking for trouble by consuming caffeine late in the day. If you smoke, then try and back-off as early in the day as you can. Nicotine, a stimulant, as stated before will interfere with your sleep stages. Even though alcohol is a depressant and it can assist in getting you to the front door of sleep, it can also keep you out of the deep stages in the slumber cycle that you require for rejuvenating rest. A drink or two may be okay depending upon the way your body reacts to the alcohol, but limit your intake if you have any doubts.
4. **Develop a routine.** A pre-sleep routine helps to get you in the right frame of mind for sleeping. The old saying of mind over matter certainly has relevancy when it comes to sleep. Try too hard to get to sleep and you'll lie awake for hours. On the other hand, letting your mind wander through different relaxing thoughts can put you right to sleep. Have a specific routine to warm down before retiring. Read a book or magazine, watch the tube, take about ten minutes to stretch your limbs, lay your

clothes out for the next day, converse with your spouse about semi-meaningless topics or do anything that will relax you and take your mind off of potentially stressful areas of concern. This is not the time to discuss your financial plights, your kid's future, or your mother in law. Yoga, hot chocolate or watching Leno can all help. It is crucial for you to get into the right frame of mind without trying too hard. It also helps to go to bed and wake up at the same time each and every day of the week. Huge importance! It's extremely important to establish a routine for your body to adjust to in order to form good habits. Routine, routine, routine!!!

5. **Bedrooms are for sleeping.** Your bedroom should have one use and one use only; and that is for sleeping . . . okay, maybe two uses, but only two! Don't use your room as a center of entertainment, for the kids to hang out in, as an office, hobby room or a place to rebuild your old motorcycle. You need to associate your bedroom with sleep and not much else. Allowing *anything* else in your bedroom will give your mind an excuse to wander in the wrong areas. Again, the brain can project powerful control over your conscious and subconscious activities, and this is an area that you can exert at least some control over your mental center. Do not underestimate the power of your brain to control your sleep functions.
6. **Forgedaboudit!** Don't discuss stress trigger topics before going to, or while in bed. (An example would be anything to do with your offspring!) If you have things that need to be discussed, please take care of them early in the evening, not while brushing your teeth before hopping in the sack. It's not very productive and will sidetrack your sleep process. Thinking is the last thing you want to do when your head hits that pillow.
7. **Stuffed.** Don't stuff or starve yourself too close to bedtime. Too much liquid or food in your belly can either give you an upset stomach or make you uncomfortable upon retiring. Besides,

you don't need any more excuses to get up in the middle of the night. On the opposite side, don't go to bed very hungry. You'll have food and not sleep on your mind. Limiting your amount of food intake in the evening can also help the diet process by allowing your stomach to shrink somewhat while you sleep. The same holds true for liquids-not much before bedtime. Try and limit food and drink intake several hours before bedtime. Don't eat for at least three hours and stop drinking an hour or two before retiring and you should be okay. If you must eat, do so lightly. Cherries have a rather high amount of melatonin, a substance manufactured in your brain to help you sleep and may not be a bad food to try. Better yet, cherry juice has ten times the concentration of melatonin that the fruit itself. Don't drink too much or you'll end up taking too many trips to the bathroom while consuming too many calories.

8. **Address chronic pain.** Chronic pain and/or depression will do more damage to the slumber process than just about any other factor. If you suffer constant joint or muscle aches, have been diagnosed with any type of depression or even feel you may be suffering an abnormal amount of anxiety, then the chances are good that those factors are affecting your quality of sleep. If you have aches and pains during the day, chances are that they are affecting you during your sleep. The pain can awaken you when it gets severe enough, which could be several times nightly, even if you don't remember. The depression or mental problems can keep you from obtaining and staying asleep. Both types of problems need to be addressed. Unfortunately both will probably have to be taken care of by a professional. There are many fixes for chronic pain. The first is identifying the actual problem, which may involve a visit to a doctor to determine if you have arthritis or just a particular joint or muscle tear or pull. This is crucial because you don't want to do a blind treatment that may not fix or relieve the problem. See a doctor, but in the meantime find some way to relieve the pain

with stretching, hot or cold presses, over-the-counter painkillers, plus exercise. Exercise is crucial to strengthening and relieving those muscles. You need to be on a regular workout program. The sleep gods will thank you. I wish that I could help with the emotional problems, but the only assistance I can offer is that you are not alone. As mentioned before, there are huge numbers of people in this country who have experienced at least some degree of trauma or emotional instability for a variety of reasons. Most of the time they go undiagnosed, quite often until it's too late. Don't be shy or embarrassed; just seek help. There is one suggestion though and that is to try a natural approach with exercise, supplements, counseling sessions, etc. Stay away from a chemical band-aid that will only cause other problems later and may interfere with your precious sleep.

9. **Exercise regularly.** Regular exercise is a great help. We have discussed the hormone serotonin that is released when exercising which will help relax your body. It will also exhaust your muscles, relieve tension, give you an outlet for your excess energy and will make you feel good about yourself. The only caveat is not to do heavy exercise within a couple of hours of your bedtime — you will be too wound up to sleep. Exercise will be discussed in a chapter of its own but is important to mention here.
10. **Give up and get up!** If it ain't happening, get up. If sleep doesn't come within fifteen to thirty minutes, then you're wasting your time. Get up and go mow the yard . . . just kidding. You'll wake the neighbors! Get up and read, watch TV, do some very light and meaningless chores or just something that is sure to bore you to death until you're ready to get back to sleep. Studies have shown that tossing and turning does you no good and will actually delay your slumber if you stay there, so get something done instead. There is plenty of lousy late-night television to lull you right to sleep.

Severe Chronic Insomnia

This section is reserved for those of you who are way past getting good rest even after following the above-mentioned steps. If you've been having a horrible experience in trying to get to sleep for a long time and apnea has been ruled out, these guidelines may help, but you may need to go to the next level by going to war against the monster that's keeping you awake. In the book, *Desperately Seeking Snoozin'* (great name for a book), by John Wiedman, he discovered a method that helped him tremendously. You may think you have sleep problems, but I doubt seriously that they even come close to what this poor man went through. He got plenty of on-the-job training for the material used in his book. **He used most of our top ten sleep suggestions with some changes.**

First, establish the time that you must wake up every morning. Then determine the absolute minimum amount of sleep you feel that you need to function properly the next day. It is crucial that you do this. Do not use the amount of sleep you would *like* to have, but the hours needed, at a minimum, to make it through tomorrow. Subtract that from your wake up time to determine when you go to sleep. If that time happens to be 12:30 AM, do not retire before that time!!! Do all you can to stay awake until then without using any caffeine or other stimulating activities. **The idea is that you going to be so damn tired by the time you actually get into bed that the quality of sleep that you will get will be much better.** You won't toss and turn as much, nor will you be able to stay awake either.

After several nights of better quality rest, then slowly back up the time that you enter the bed in order to increase the amount of sleep that you get. I know it sounds like an insane way to approach sleep problems, but it seems to work. Part of this strategy is to develop healthy habits by rebooting your internal time clock, among other things. If your problems are severe, then read this very informative book.

Sleep Conclusions

The importance of a good night's sleep cannot be underestimated. Your body absolutely needs rest to rebuild itself at the cellular level. Deep sleep is when your body releases growth hormones that assist in repairing the damage done throughout the day, the brain resets itself and your immune system is retooled. You cannot function properly without the correct amount of restful sleep each and every night.

Sleep is a habit. Your habit may be good or it may be terrible. It's important to attack any health problems with a specific plan and sleep is no different. First determine if you have any medical conditions that can affect sleep that need to be addressed. Next get rid of any distractions that are keeping your ever so powerful mind from the job at hand and use our top ten sleep suggestions to make it easier to obtain blissful snoozing.

Most all diseases and bodily deteriorations happen as a result of cellular breakdown of some sort. Sleep is the one area that can stop the degradation, thus keeping your cells from dying off. Conquer the sleep monster and your life will improve dramatically without even doing anything else, plus you will live longer to boot!

Step 3:

Use It or Lose It

Exercise. You had to know this was going to be included in your program somewhere. There's not a health plan in the world worth its salt that doesn't contain exercise as an integral part of its foundation, and this is no exception. It is, without a doubt, *as* crucial as *any* item on our ten-step program. You cannot hope to obtain or maintain a decent level of long-term health without it. You may have gotten away with being a couch potato up till now, but there is no avoiding it anymore.

On the other hand, this is not an exercise book. If it were, it would be twice as long with double the chapters devoted to many different types of exercise and plenty of explanations as to why working out is important for you. We'll try to concentrate our limited space and your time on exactly why you should exercise, some general programs to get you started, and we'll throw in a few pointers and tidbits of information to make it more interesting.

For those of you who despise exercising and see it as a huge chore, (apparently there are plenty of you) a recent government report showed that seven out of ten adults do not exercise on a regular basis. That's only twenty minutes of vigorous activities three times a week! A pathetic statistic given the benefits of an exercise program.

Maybe you are looking at the whole concept of getting sweaty in the wrong context. There was an interesting perspective on exercising offered by Leslie Garcia, who wrote fifty-two helpful health tips for the new year (2003) in the *Dallas Morning News.* She wrote, *"Consider the ability to exercise a gift, not an obligation. How wonderful to have legs that can walk, arms that can lift even a 1-pound free weight."* I'm sure Christopher Reeves, among others, has that perspective, and it may not be a bad way for you to look at exercising either.

The average adult loses five pounds of muscle mass every decade after reaching the age of forty-five! If you live to be 110, all that will be left of you will be a blob of fat, some small brittle bones and that undigested burrito left in your belly from 1987. If you add exercise to your daily routine, you can at least stall if not reverse the depletion of your muscular system. Add exercise to your life and by the time you reach *old* age, not only will you be chasing nurses around your ward, you'll still be pulling down twenty rebounds a game, *and* will run circles around your great-grandkids. Okay, maybe a small stretch. You'll probably be lucky to get eight to ten rebounds per game coming off the bench, and you'll probably chase anything that you can catch (like maybe a mannequin in the window of The Gap).

"I guess I have to keep in shape as I get older,
but I don't like to work out.
Whenever I get the urge to exercise,
I lie down until it passes." –Al Pacino

Why exercise?

Losing muscle mass, as noted earlier, can spell big-time trouble. It can lead to back problems including curvature of the spine, weight gain, fatigue, and a whole array of ailments and discomforts that can be avoided or at least delayed by implementing a regular exercise program. You'll notice the key word here is "regular." Regular, for this example, can be defined as "at least three times a week, each and every week throughout the remainder of your life." At the beginning of this book we talked about making a change in your lifestyle and noted that your "good health" would require a commitment ***from you, by you, and for you.*** Now is the time for that commitment, and the area that can make the biggest and most noticeable change in the way you look and feel is exercise. There is no beating around the proverbial bush. It will take a rather large commitment of your time and effort. In fact, it's quite easy to say that out of all the steps outlined in this program, exercise is the one area that will demand the most of you. There will be times when you don't feel like working out or don't think you have the time, and you will just try and come up with some excuse not to get out of bed or off your butt. Your inner demons will test your resolve. Your dedication to this program and your health will be tested time and time again. Of course, it is up to you and only you to stay on the path. Exercise by itself won't improve your health entirely, but it is one of the main ingredients absolutely necessary to put you on that road to a new you.

I would have liked to tell you that there is, or will be, a pill that will make exercise obsolete, but that will never, ever happen. We would all much prefer a Caribbean beach and pinã coladas instead of the gym, but first you will need exercise to get you looking good before you can venture into the hot sand without scaring off a group of teenagers. If one of those teenagers happen to be related to you, it's better to scare them off by embarrassing them with something you say than by the appearance of your body.

Preserving your muscular structure is certainly not the only benefit of incorporating exercise into your daily life. Many other advantages are plentiful. For instance, diabetes can be avoided by a regular exercise regime and proper diet. When you exercise, your body fuels itself by taking glucose out of your blood to use for that particular activity, allowing your system to regulate glucose more efficiently. In diabetes, the pancreas, which releases insulin into your bloodstream to regulate blood sugar levels eventually wears out from years of shoving simple sugars into your blood thereby continually spiking your blood sugar level. Exercise and a proper diet can help alleviate and prevent this horrible disease.

The Blues

Exercise not only releases serotonin, dopamine and other naturally occurring beneficial hormones into your body that can help curb depression and other psychological disorders, it will inevitably make you feel better about yourself, thus adding a great mental advantage to everything you do. Duke University researchers found that exercise works at least as well as a major prescription drug in treating clinical depression! (They failed to mention that it's usually a lot less expensive and has no side effects.) Part of the findings of this study suggested that their patients gained a sense of control over their lives that drugs couldn't match. Not only did the depression go away, it stayed gone, too. Another benefit of the serotonin release is the positive effect that it has on rest and sleep, the importance of this cannot be stated enough.

Heart Friendly

Would you like to reduce your risk of a stroke or heart attack? Dumb question. Working out reduces your blood pressure, raises the level of HDL cholesterol (the good kind), and increases the strength of your heart muscles. Translation? **You can cut your risk**

in these areas by 50%! It doesn't take much. Women over the age of 45 whose only form of exercise was to walk for one hour a week halved their risk of coronary artery disease according to a study of nearly 40,000 women. Men had similar results in another study. Even though one hour is not enough to make a difference in other areas of your health, the fact that it can influence your risk of heart disease by so much for so little effort is short of amazing.

Joint Pain/Cancer fighter

Exercise can significantly reduce the pain caused by arthritis by keeping muscles and joints loose, flexible and strong. Exercise, to arthritis, is like WD-40 is to squeaky metal parts in your car.

Not surprisingly, the American Cancer Society has added regular exercise to its list of preventative measures to stop cancer, as **they determined that unfit men were three times more likely to die from cancer than physically fit men! Not to discriminate, they also discovered that sedentary women had sixteen times the cancer death rate than women who were in good physical condition!**

Chronic Conditions

For those of you who are already suffering from any chronic illness, studies have also found that a regular exercise program can have a profound effect on your well-being. **It has recently been shown to have a positive effect on chronic inflammation, a major indicator of many different ailments including cancers of all types and heart disease.** Exercise, beyond anything else, is energizing and empowering, and it gives you at least some control over your predicament. Even your automobile wasn't made to just sit in a garage. It also needs to be used. It does not have the ability to regenerate itself as you do, but it, too, will seize up if not exercised.

"I like long walks, especially when they are taken by people that annoy me." –Anonymous

WHAT'S IT GOING TO TAKE?

If you are not going to work out at least three times a week then you will not get the benefits you need to overcome forty or so years of sitting on your couch eating Twinkies and watching reruns of *The Andy Griffith Show!* You're probably thinking, "I don't have the time! I have two kids, two jobs and too many other commitments to make more time for some stupid exercise program." Sorry, but that doesn't cut the proverbial mustard! *Everyone on this planet has the same amount of time each and every day, and there are plenty of people who do a whole lot more than you and I, and they still have time to exercise regularly.* If the President of the United States has time to jog in the morning and play around with the hired help in the afternoon, then certainly you can get off your ever-expanding butt and do something for yourself each and every day.

Exercising is actually a very selfish activity. It's time that you spend on yourself and generally benefits nobody else. It is for the betterment of you. Not directly for your spouse or kids. Not for your best friend or your parents. It benefits you, but as has been mentioned, it indirectly benefits everyone around you.

So remember, selfishness can be a good thing though. How will you have the energy to put into your friends, spouse and family if getting through the day, by itself, is a struggle? **If you don't take care of yourself, then how can you take care of anybody else? Do you really want to burden your children with the job of having to take care of you later in life, just because you didn't take care of yourself now?** Do you want them to have to help you in and out of a wheelchair because you didn't take your health seriously.

The amount of time you spend working out will reap benefits way beyond the effort you put into it. Playing with your grandkids, seeing them graduate, spending extra quality time with your loved ones, keeping up with the neighbor kids and having the energy to make the most of traveling and your retirement. **Not being confined to a wheelchair and just plain enjoying life are in your reach and should not be taken for granted. A lot of things can happen between now and senility. There are no guarantees that you will be able to care for yourself ten to fifteen years from now, unless you begin taking care of yourself immediately.** An ongoing exercise program will: make you stronger, beef up your skeletal structure, improve you immune system, increase the blood flow to your brain thus staving off diseases such as Alzheimer's, lower your blood pressure and cholesterol, and reduce the risk of heart disease, etc. . . . It's a win-win proposition. Don't have any regrets later — get off your butt now!

SQUEEZE PLAY

Let's discuss the time you say you don't have. Do you have a lunch hour at work? Eat at your desk after a workout! Is there a gym in your building? Use it, and not the excuse of messing up your hair because of the workout. Nobody really cares what your hair looks like. They are too busy worrying about how they look. Do you work in or near a high-rise building? If so, climbing steps is one of the best exercises that you can undertake (take it easy though, especially if your knees are toast, and work your way up very slowly increasing the number of flights climbed weekly. As with *any* exercise program, if you have knee problems, check with your doctor first.)

At least you can walk during your lunch hour. Go through your downtown area, a nearby mall (no shopping allowed) or around your office building or plant. Get some friends to go with you and make it more fun. If you have a flexible work schedule and environment, then you have absolutely no excuse. Join the YMCA or a convenient club. Be creative. You don't need a gym to get your heart pumping. (Seeing a picture of Brad Pitt doesn't count.) A jump rope, some dumbbells, a couple of chairs or phone books, a bench, some stairs, a parking garage, an indoor mall, some hills behind your home or just staying one step ahead of the IRS can give you *all* the exercise you need.

What about after work? Get your family to participate by walking, hiking, riding bikes or going to the gym with you. I know . . . you're too tired after work. That's the whole reason to workout in the first place! The workout will energize you (eventually), and you will actually look forward to your "me-time". Buy a workout video and make a fool of yourself in front of the tube. Enjoy! Yes, you too can look like Richard Simmons! Oh boy . . .

We all have things that come up during the day making it difficult to work out on a regular basis. Because of that, there is one time in the day that you *don't* have any excuses and that is early in the morning *before* going to work. Yeah, that means resetting your alarm. It may mean getting up a lot earlier than you wish. That can be very tough in the beginning, but you will get used to the early alarm if you take intelligent precautions like going to bed earlier and being prepared for the activity, laying out the clothes that you will need the night before, etc. The exercise will energize your day. There are some important physiological advantages to morning exercise. One, morning workouts burn more body fat because insulin levels are steadier at that time of the morning. It also elevates your metabolism for the entire day, allowing you to churn away more calories than otherwise, and it has been found to make you feel more relaxed, too. Getting your workout over early frees up the rest of your day allowing you time enough to do the things that are important to you like giving your cat a bath, organizing your silverware drawer, chatting with your mother-in-law or painting the outside of your home, to name a few!

TOP TEN REASONS TO EXERCISE

Here's a look at the ten best reasons to get on a regular exercise program and better your life.

10. You'll be able to run circles around your kids again.
9. You'll be able to hang out longer at the office water cooler without tiring.
8. Your letter jacket will fit again.
7. Your friends will call you "Buff" or "Stud."
6. Stronger arms means being able to carry more cases of beer.
5. Hollywood will call.
4. People will like you more because you're "cool" now.
3. Just let that other team's parent pick on your kid.
2. Your golf handicap will be cut in half (just playing 9 holes helps too).
1. And the number one reason for exercising is......

SEX, SEX AND MORE SEX!

Let's hope your partner has been exercising, too.

Whoops, wrong list.........there are so many ***real*** reason to hit the gym, but we'll go over some of the most important ones again and in more detail in order to scare the crap out of you, forcing you to take up a new lifestyle whether you like it or not. (This program is not above using intimidation in order to reach the goal of getting you off of your can). Let's discuss the *other* top ten list of reasons to exercise.

1. **Adult onset (or type 2) diabetes:** In the last decade alone, this form of diabetes has increased tremendously in the U.S. due mainly to a decrease in exercise *and* a lousy diet. It is found

mainly, but not exclusively, in obese people. We didn't used to see this horrendous disease in people under fifty years of age, but now we are increasingly seeing it in people as young as thirty and sometimes in teenagers! Unfortunately, there are even cases of toddlers, usually obese, contracting this horrible disease.

You do not want this disease . . . diabetes triples the risk of heart attacks, it is the leading cause of blindness in people between twenty and sixty-five. It's also a major reason for kidney failure and leg amputations! You will more than likely die earlier than necessary if you contract this horrible disease . . . On top of these facts, if you *do* contract it, which by the way is virtually incurable today, the management of this is a royal pain in the butt! Your diet will be much more restrictive than ever before and you'll have to monitor your blood sugar level several times a day by pricking your fingers to test the blood sugar level in your body at that moment. Not a fun way to live, but surely a quick way to die! In fact, if contracted in your teenage years, it will take up to twenty-seven years off your life.

Without proper exercise or good dietary habits, Type 2 Diabetes occurs when your pancreas quits making enough insulin and/or your body becomes insulin resistant, meaning your system cannot make proper use of the hormone, which is absolutely required for cellular metabolism. Your system uses insulin to assist in converting the junk you call food that enters your body into glucose and enables that (sugar) to go into each and every cell to be used as fuel. The pancreas (which makes the insulin) tries to compensate for this constant spiking of your blood sugar level by making more and more of this hormone. Eventually the insulin producing cells just plain wear out and therein lies the problem. Basically, if not corrected, every cell in your body is starved to death, the oxygen rich organs such as your eyes and heart go first. Your life will forever change.

This is not something you want to deal with after the fact. Get off your butt, lose weight and greatly reduce your possibility of contracting diabetes by exercising! **Don't think that it can't happen to you because it can. Having a sedentary lifestyle combined with a bad diet can be deadly.** Diabetes is caused by the continued abuse of your system and because of this fact there will never be a drug invented to completely take care of this hideous disease. Surprisingly, regular exercise has been shown to have more of an impact on the threat of diabetes than even your diet.

2. Contracting diabetes, by itself, *should* be reason enough to exercise. However, if you need more convincing, the next major reason is to **relieve, prevent or retard the development of several forms of arthritis.** Arthritis is simply an inflammation of one or more joints characterized by swelling, pain, stiffness and immobility of that particular area. Almost fifty million people in the U.S. suffer from this ailment. There are many different types including: rheumatoid arthritis, osteoarthritis, and gout. Rheumatoid arthritis is generally found in the joints of the hands, feet, hips and shoulders. The severity can be wide, ranging from a minor inconvenience to a crippling disability. The symptoms can sometimes go into remission. Joint replacement is not out of the realm of possibilities. Osteoarthritis, the most common of this class of disease, is associated mainly with the joint cartilage and is recognized by the narrowing of the joint space due to the loss of that cartilage. This occurs usually in later life and also can be crippling. Gout, which has to do with a defect in uric acid metabolism affecting the joints, can also be very, very painful, and destructive in nature. (A proper diet may especially help keep gout in check.)

   Guess what? **A regular exercise program can beat this crippling monster!** If you run your automobile on a regular basis, you'll keep the metal and moving parts from seizing or rusting out. The same applies to your body. You have to keep your joints moving, maintain flexibility and be strong enough to hold your body upright in a proper posture. Exercise will cause you to run a lot of blood through your system, flushing out any toxic build-up and continually nourishing all of your cells. Adding resistance training to your regular program stresses the muscles, tendons and ligaments supporting the bones, which stimulates bone growth. **We're talking about a real "quality of life" issue when dealing with the inevitability of having some form of arthritis as we age.** Be pro-active and prevent it from happening in the first place. If you are unfortunate enough to have it now, then reduce its severity through regular exercise. You don't want to look like Quasimoto, do you?

3. The next reason to exercise should be an obvious one. The majority of Americans at one time or another have suffered from **back pain.** It has caused them to miss work along with having to endure the misery and limitations caused by many different problems. Having to stay in bed, not playing with the little ones, experiencing discomfort sitting or standing, trouble sleeping and suffering from headaches are all problems associated with back pain.

   To help prevent or relieve back discomfort you need to build up the muscles between your upper thighs and neck, front and back by using a combination of resistance exercises and aerobic training. By making these muscles stronger it becomes easier to hold yourself upright and will take unneeded pressure off sensitive areas along your spine. A stronger torso makes a healthier back. Again, be proactive and prevent problems before they happen. The areas to concentrate on include: your hip area, abdominal muscles, shoulders, neck and of course your back muscles. By strengthening all of them, pressure will be taken off of the spine itself causing less "spasming" of the muscles and will give you a better quality of life. You can't just do sit-ups and assume that is all that you need. Sit-ups, pushups, shoulder shrugs, rowing, side bends and leg raises are just some of the exercises that you can incorporate into your regime to go along with walking, jogging, swimming or bicycling. Incidentally, doctors used to recommend bed rest for back problems. Not anymore. Now they want you to get off your derrière and at least exercise moderately. By moving continuously, the increased blood flow will help speed the recovery and will also keep your back muscles from atrophying, which is one of the worst things that can happen. **The reduction in pain through exercise has also been shown to be greater than using painkillers.**

4. **Anxiety and depression,** unfortunately, are as much a part of today's society as obnoxious talk show hosts. These maladies can be eliminated or at least kept to a minimum by exercising, which raises the level of a brain chemical called serotonin. This chemical, one of the most important ones produced by your body, will literally help you feel better. Most of the successful anti-depression medicines on the market today affect the serotonin levels in your brain. That is all they do! On the other hand, exercise also lowers the level of adrenaline, which can cause symptoms associated with depression. Being in less discomfort, having more energy, and the ability to sleep better also help your mental well-being, as does being stronger, not feeling as tired, having good physical health, looking more attractive and your clothes fitting better all contribute to your positive mental well being. **It is a crime that regular exercise is not prescribed for depression by our medical community.** Think of how much money we could save and how many side effects could be avoided by eliminating anti-depressants from our lives and treating depression with exercise.
5. **Your heart and lungs** are assisted in their normal operation by muscles, and of course exercising builds up the strength of these most important organs. Your poor overworked heart pumps more than a gallon of blood a minute and up to 2000 gallons a day! You will enjoy a lower, more efficient pulse rate, a healthier blood pressure level, and by exercising regularly will greatly lower your risk of heart disease and stroke. This should be of no surprise to you since there have been hundreds of studies for several decades showing the health benefits to your respiratory system by a regular exercise routine. For this particular benefit, the minimum you need to do is walk briskly four to five times a week for thirty to forty-five minutes each time and you'll

reap the rewards without any other method of exercise!

One study showed that people who walked only one and one-half miles daily had half the heart attack risk than those that only walked half of a mile. One and a half miles only takes about twenty-five minutes depending on your pace. Although this isn't enough exercise for your total health program, hopefully you'll see the power of exercising as it relates to your overall well-being.

Exercise (and a proper diet) also reduces a specific chronic inflammation deep within the recesses of your blood vessels that **has recently been shown to be the single most powerful trigger of heart attacks. This is huge news. These painless, and thus silent irritations are apparently worse on your circulatory system than elevated cholesterol!** (This inflammation can be measured with a simple blood test that checks for C-reactive protein [CRP].) Add the use of proper natural anti-inflammatory supplements, even aspirin if you must, plus exercise and you'll knock these silent killers out of your blood supply system.

6. **Most everyone wishes to lose weight** and there is no better way than working out on a regular basis (the exceptions being; wiring your mouth shut, being stranded on a desert island [or is that a dessert isle?], getting divorced or living with your in-laws!). So how does this work? There are two ways to lose weight: one, through the act of exercise itself. After burning 3500 more calories than you have consumed, you will have lost one pound. (It's a lot easier putting weight on than taking it off, isn't it?) Secondly, through another benefit of your exercise program, your base metabolic rate (BMR) increases after exercising and continues for some time after that. It takes energy to break down and rebuild muscle cells and this process is what burns the excess calories. In other word, while you stand, walk, work, talk or even sleep after exercising you are burning more calories than you would if you had not exercised. This is especially true after a resistance type of workout. So don't be

disappointed at the realization that your workout only burned 'x' number of calories: you'll continue to burn extra ones for a long time. This is especially important since our metabolic rate decreases as we get older even if we reduce the intake of food and is one of the main reasons we put on weight as we age.

7. Another benefit of idolizing Richard Simmons is your **ability to sleep better.** As we have discussed previously, restful sleep is a huge problem as we age and conquering it is much easier with exercise. In addition to exhausting your muscles, you release hormones that relax you naturally. It also serves as a diversion from your everyday problems by taking your mind off of problems and gives you a sense of accomplishment.
8. Do you plan on having any **major traumas** like a bad car wreck or major surgery? Of course not. Who knows what is going to happen tomorrow, next week or next year? By being in shape now, you'll recover better and quicker than you would otherwise, if you should happen to be put in some unfortunate situation. **The chance of having major surgery increases with age and recovery is a lot quicker if you are healthier than otherwise, so it pays to put in the time now on that treadmill.** Talk about being in control! Now that's really being prepared for life's twists and turns!
9. **Glaucoma** is a condition in which a loss of vision occurs because of abnormally high pressure in the eyes. As we age the possibility of this happening increases. Exercising helps in the prevention of this disease. Even though glaucoma is treatable by surgery, eye drops, and other methods, why bother putting yourself though the discomfort or misery of treatment when exercising is available to help prevent it now?
10. Last, but certainly not least, exercise may reduce the risk of **impotence!** Even walking at little as two miles a day (easy to do) can reduce your chances of getting "erectile dysfunction" by 50%. (I think its safe to assume that we're talking to the male population here, but women have a stake here also!) Researchers from the New England Research Institute believe

that since exercise fights vascular diseases, the increased blood flow keeps those particular arteries healthy and clear of problems. The more exercise the men on this study did, the lower the chances were that they would develop impotence. Before you get on your treadmill and attempt to run for three straight weeks without stopping, you may want to slow down and not worry too much about this. This particular problem will take care of itself while you are taking better care of yourself.

11. Whoops, appears that I miscounted. There are more than ten good reasons to work out. A study released from Duke University by Dr. William E. Kraus reveals a new **relationship between exercise and cholesterol.** While only rigorous exercise can increase your HDL (good) level, most exercise, by itself, has little effect on cholesterol as a whole. This interesting research demonstrated that even modest levels of exercise do not change the overall numbers, but alter the size and density of cholesterol-carrying proteins so that they cause less damage to your circulatory system. Basically, exercising thins out the number of cholesterol particles that are capable of doing damage. Moderate exercise alone will not reduce the overall level of cholesterol, but will keep it from causing problems to your cardiovascular system. Another great reason to hit the gym.
12. Here's still another great reason to exercise: **Osteoporosis can be greatly stalled or even prevented by regular weight-bearing exercises.** The rebuilding of your bones is basically the same as rebuilding your muscles. If you don't use them, then you'll lose them! Osteoporosis is completely unnecessary. Eat some weights and lift a little calcium to keep your bones strong. (Was that backwards?)

Although there are several other reasons to exercise, these ten . . . I mean twelve, are the most important. No really! That's it! No more. Twelve benefits are more than enough.

What are those twelve reasons again?

1. To prevent diabetes.
2. To halt arthritis.
3. To prevent or relieve back pain.
4. To eliminate or minimize depression.
5. To strengthen your heart and lungs.
6. To lose weight.
7. To sleep better.
8. To strengthen you against future trauma or illness.
9. To prevent glaucoma.
10. To eliminate impotence.
11. To lower cholesterol.
12. To stop or even reverse osteoporosis.

"My grandmother started walking 5 miles a day when she was 60. She is now 87 and we don't have a clue where she is."

–Anonymous

Nuts and Bolts

Okay, now that we have established that an exercise program as a worthwhile and critical step to your continued health, what kind of exercise should you do and how often do you participate? The short answer is: any kind you can and as often as is possible. However, let's get a little more specific and divide your program into two categories.

Some of you may already be exercising. Wonderful! You may be walking, jogging, biking, swimming, playing tennis or golf, working in your yard, and if you're lucky, getting lucky as well. If you are already physically active, then some fine-tuning may be all that you need.

It's important to combine both resistance *and* aerobic forms of exercise into one complete program. Weight training and other forms of resistance training strengthen your muscles and bones, help your posture, improve your looks, and cause you to burn more calories during periods of inactivity. Surprising recent data shows that resistance training is more important than aerobic exercise as you age. That does not mean that you can quit walking or riding a bike. It only means that you need to put as much emphasis on resistant training as your time allows.

Aerobic exercise (walking, running, swimming, bicycling, etc.) helps your endurance, overall strength in several muscle groups including your heart and lungs, and contributes to the overall health of your system. It is imperative, and much more fun, to have a little variety in your routine, mixing several different activities together. You will stick with it longer, and it will improve your overall coordination to boot.

On a weekly basis, ideally, you should be doing two to three days of resistance training and four to five days of aerobic activity. "Wait a minute," you say. "Doing the math totals up to eight days per week!" Yeah, so what? Don't you have eight days in your week? Actually, by combining some activities together you can get *both* types of exercises into one workout. The key to aerobic training is to get your heart rate up for an extended period of time, and it really doesn't matter how it gets there. If you're working on weight machines and can move from station to station quickly, and not resting along the way, then you may get both types of exercises done. (If you can have a pleasant conversation the entire time that you're lifting, then you're probably not getting much of an aerobic workout.) Plus, if you get up early in the morning and do something like walking, there is no reason why you can't lift weights in the afternoon or evening of the same day. If swimming laps or running fairly long distances is a part of your routine then you may be able to also take credit for both types of exercise, especially since both are very strenuous workouts. However, swimming doesn't put enough resistance on your bone structure, so you'll more than likely have to lift also.

I can hear the excuse train approaching . . too many days, too much time, and too much money! You can get this done in as few as four days, five is highly doable and ideal. Resting your body and letting it recover is also crucial. Don't do strenuous resistance exercises every day of the week. Give your poor muscle cells a chance to get stronger. We are not "Super" men and women. Remember that variety is also important. Resting is just as important as the exercise itself.

Taking time out of your day to do something for yourself should not be avoided. This is the part of the commitment that we discussed earlier. Either wake up early in the morning, use your lunch hour, or find time in the evening. "Just do it." (Hey, I think I'll copyright that phrase!)

"I don't exercise at all. If God meant us to touch our toes, he would have put them further up our body." –My wife

THE MONEY PITS

The best and last argument Americans use against exercising is the money it can cost for the equipment or the gym membership. Of course it can be very expensive to buy a ton of equipment or join a fancy gym. Go ahead and spend the money if you wish. If not, then consider the alternatives.

There are several things you can do right from your home that are great exercises but don't cost much money. Yes, you are correct in assuming that we'll talk about ten examples that don't cost much, if anything at all.

The Top Ten Exercises Not Costing an Arm and a Leg:

1. Exercise videos. Any of them! All that you need is a TV, VCR and a video tape you can even check out at the library, buy at any used book store or find cheap at Wal-Mart. Best of all, you can make a complete idiot of yourself and nobody ever has to know! (Unless you have neighbors living below you!) Thirty to sixty minutes of this and you've got an excellent aerobic exercise.
2. Walking or running shoes. Put them on, grab your watch and a pair of dumbbells. (No, not your sister's kids! The other ones!) About five to ten pounds each will be sufficient to increase the benefits of a long quick walk. Suck in your gut, throw your shoulders back and walk a fast pace of about three to four miles per hour if you can. Do this for at least thirty minutes, concentrate on your breathing, and the long term benefits will be incredible not to mention the short-term toning that will take place. Also, do us all a favor. Don't walk down the street flailing your arms everywhere like you're drowning in a pool of hot oil . . . you'll embarrass the rest of us! Walking normal will suffice. If you can power walk five days a week and add two to three days of weights (skip a day or two in between the weight training), you'll be set! Remember, this isn't meant to be a stroll in the park. Keep it moving quickly.
3. Climb stairs, hike hills or walk up a parking garage. Do you live in a high rise? Is your part of the world hilly? If you can take advantage of gravity instead of *it* taking advantage of you, you will get one of the best workouts available. Again, if your knees are shot, check with your doctor first and take it easy.
4. Mow the yard! Save the money you're paying the neighbor kid, get a non self-propelled mower and take off. In the summer, you can have a very good excuse for mowing twice a week if you want. Your lawn will love that! When pushing the mower, put the handle against your hips and let your legs do most of

the pushing. (If you have a bad neck or back, the unnatural angle of the pushing motion puts a strain on your back.) This is great exercise and can save you a ton of money. Best of all, this is an activity that both men and women can do. Don't look at me that way, ladies . . . just trying to give you equal time!

5. Jump rope. Chances are you can't do three minutes of this fantastic boxer's routine. Neither can your kids, so don't worry. You probably don't want to center your complete program around this, but it can serve to break the boredom at times and help you with your balance.
6. Dumbbells. You can purchase good ones for about fifty cents per pound and you'll need three to four different pairs of them. For women- three, eight, twelve and fifteen pounds each should suffice. For men- eight, twelve, fifteen and twenty-five will probably do. Obviously, this is just a range. You may find that others work better. If you can afford a flat workout bench (approx. $100), you can fashion a great home-based workout using these, a pair of folding chairs for dips, phone books for pushups and a basketball to work out your gut. You don't ever have to leave your beautiful home!
7. Chin-up bar. It can be purchased inexpensively at any sporting goods store and is great for chin-ups, pull-ups, leg- raises (great for your gut), and stretching. You can also make your own with a piece of sturdy metal. Make sure that whichever one you use is anchored to studs in the wall. (That's so you don't fall on your head like I did several years ago while hanging upside down in a pair of inversion boots! Landed right on my head and bounced! That was lots of fun and probably explains much of my present behavior.)
8. Bicycle. Most everyone has a bike. Use it. If the weather doesn't cooperate, you can purchase a stand to put it on so you can put in several miles and minutes in your garage or living room. Make sure it is comfortable and fits your now-shrinking butt properly.
9. Work in the yard. You shouldn't be surprised to learn that pulling weeds, planting flowers, raking leaves, shoveling snow

and digging holes can be hard work and will burn tons of calories. Again, if you have back problems, take it easy. Don't lift bags of dirt, mulch, fertilizer or anything heavy unless you keep it very close to your body. Lift with your legs, not your back.

10. Clean the house. No, scrub it. Spend several hours giving it a polish and you'll accomplish more than just exercise. Having the maid or your spouse doing the work doesn't count. Do it yourself, including the vacuuming (remember, keep the vacuum close to your body to avoid torso strain).

Are we running out of excuses yet? If not, we haven't even talked about joining a health club, your local YMCA, city recreation center, church, school or apartment facility, any of which has plenty of equipment to keep you sweating, grunting and groaning. There are personal trainers and plenty of people to help get you started regardless of your age or degree of fitness. You are not alone. There are thousands of people daily that start exercising for the first time in their lives, unfortunately there are just as many that stop. Don't be a quitter. By the way, if you have some physical ailment, any money that you spend exercising may be tax deductible! Check with your CPA. Make sure that you use the Enron-trained accountants for the best results!

"I joined a health club last year, spent about $400. Haven't lost a pound. Apparently you have to show up."
-Anonymous. (You can take credit for this one!)

Make it work

Two or three times weekly of a resistance program is easy to do. Choose a program that works for you depending on your likes, dislikes, time, and convenience. If you work close to a health club or YMCA and can work it in, then this will be really do-able. If you can't stand to be seen with little clothing on by perfect strangers, then maybe a home routine is best. Whatever works for you will give you the best results, since you'll be more apt to stick with it if it is a setup that you enjoy. **The biggest deterrent to your success is you. Not your family, not your work, not your religion and certainly not Father Time.** Just get it done. Your muscles don't care whether you use $10,000 worth of equipment or a pair of telephone books. They will not discriminate. **However, the reason that we have hundreds of different choices in exercise equipment and regimes is because of the inherent trait in human beings to look for excuses *not* to do something *and* our gullibility when it comes to gimmicks designed to convince us to buy into a concept.** Point in case: you can work your abdominal muscles with the Ab Roller and countless other machines, wheels and crunch rotators when all you really need is to do leg lifts, sit-ups and other things you were taught in junior high! But, manufacturers are counting on you becoming bored with anything you start. They feel certain that you will quit and begin something else costing even more money . . . imagine that!

Resistance Exercise and Bone Density

Osteoporosis is the deterioration, mainly, of your load-bearing bones causing sufferers to shrink in size, hunch over and struggle with everyday life. With osteoporosis, bones become so brittle that they will break easily. Many times when you hear about older people falling down and breaking their hip, it is actually reversed. They literally break their hip and then fall! Fortunately, most bone loss is preventable and resistance exercise is the main avenue to prevent this loss.

Although your bones contain less than 15% water, they are still a living part of your body, not unlike your skin and organs. **Bone cells break down and rebuild themselves constantly. They regenerate much like any other cell in your body, just not as fast.**

Your body is constantly tearing down, building and rebuilding the internal webbing of your load-bearing bones used to support weight. **They were made to change and adapt according to the weight and stress that is placed upon them. If you are not constantly challenging them, they will get weak and brittle, not unlike your muscles going through atrophy.**

In order to strengthen and grow your bones, thus staving off osteoporosis, you have to exert enough force upon them by gradually increasing the weight they must support. (That's exactly what weight training does.) By lifting weights you actually crush some of the internal scaffolding of bone cells. This will stimulate new bone growth, making them stronger, not unlike muscle training. All the calcium, magnesium and other supplements you take will do absolutely no good in *building* bone density, unless you create demand of those minerals by your bone cells. **The biological bottom line is this: You have to lift weight or do some other resistance exercises before you will cause your bones to strengthen.** Nothing else will accomplish this. Sure, calcium, potassium and phosphorus are all important to your bones and the rest of your body's organs, but in order to help out your bone structure, there must be a demand for their services. As much as this seems to be common sense, this aspect of building bone density is not well known. However, the saying "use it or lose it" is extremely relevant here.

Whether you walk up stairs, do squats, carry boxes of books, or lift weights or children, you must stress your bone and muscle systems on a regular basis. Not only will the resistance exercises cause your bones and muscles to get stronger, you will have more energy, look better and your metabolism will be higher. A higher metabolism means that you burn off more calories and thus will have the ability to lose unwanted weight. Not a bad deal. Lifting weights, or doing any other resistance exercises is crucial in maintaining and even improving your overall health.

RESIST THIS!

Although the slight majority of your workout schedule should be centered around aerobic exercises, a minimum of two and no more than three days of your workout week should have resistance exercises as a part of them. If you are walking, running or doing other types of aerobic exercises, then three sessions of weight training are sufficient to get the job done. Lift weights, boxes, phone books, dumbbells or use any machines that mimic resistance to your bones: it doesn't really matter. But let's put a little twist to the normally accepted method of lifting to get an added benefit.

You're not striving to look like Mr. or Mrs. Universe. In fact, all you should be after is to tone things up and increase your vitality while becoming healthier. *So instead of doing the traditional two or three sets of eight to ten repetitions of each exercise using heavy weights, try this.* **Decrease the weight that you are using and do only two sets of twenty to thirty repetitions each. Don't try to lift too much and do lift slowly. It should be enough to tire your muscles sufficiently at the end of the set. This is not a contest. You aren't trying to impress anybody, nor do you care what anybody else thinks. This program is for you and your benefit only.** In order to get the bone-building benefits of resistance exercises along with energy and longevity in your waking hours, you need to lift less weight for a longer period of time. This will allow you to reach your objectives without putting unnecessary strain on your body. Many people stop exercising because of pain and discomfort. You can alleviate that problem by lifting less weight more times. You will want to lift to the point of exhausting those muscles, but no more. When you're just beginning, start out *real* slowly with less weight and build your weight and reps a little at a time. Twenty to thirty repetitions will exhaust your muscles and that is what you're after. It will build your muscular strength and endurance at the same time allowing you to shop all day at the outlet mall and carry around your entire catch without tiring. Such a deal.

WHICH MUSCLES?

Your regime should include ten to fifteen different exercises involving most of your muscles with the emphasis on your legs and torso areas, since these muscles and bones are the most relevant for your health. Don't do mainly curls and other arm exercises. They will waste your time if you don't work the other parts of your body, too. Don't worry about your arms. They'll get their share from the other exercises that you do. You can probably figure on one to two hours for the complete routine, two to three times a week. Mix that with some walking, running, swimming or biking and you'll have a well-rounded program that will give you tons of benefits.

You should work the following muscle groups in this order of priority: the back, neck and abdominal region first, legs, and then arms. **We begin with our mid-section because of all the problems we *now* have, *have* had or *will* have with our backs.** Notice that none of the choices are "will never have." Every one of you at some point in your life will have the privilege of enjoying back or neck problems. In fact, I'll make an educated guess that you already have a problem or two. Not only are these problems what they appear to be, there is a horrible snowballing effect associated with spinal problems and our overall health.

Hurt your back and making it through an entirely normal day can be a chore. It will probably exhaust you. That, in turn, will keep you from working out, will probably cause you to drink more caffeine to keep you going, and the added stress will compromise your immune system leading to colds, the flu and other ailments. Since your posture isn't the greatest with a backache, you will put added tension on different parts of your body, possibly leading to different muscle or tendon strains. You neck, knees, ankles and hamstrings are more vulnerable in these situations. Before you know it, your gym bag has mold growing in it. Although this is an over-simplification of the association of back problems to the rest of your body, they are real and you should take heed. Do not ignore or succumb to back discomfort.

Generally speaking (about backaches), your bones themselves do not generate much of the pain you are feeling. Your main discomfort comes from the muscles that have been stimulated for whatever reason and then spasm, or are pulling on a joint while tweaking nerves. This causes your muscles to pull, seize up and/or cause a world of hurt. **Over 90% of all backaches are muscle related only (muscles being stimulated by nerves, generally) and are not caused by bones cracking or moving out of joint.** That is why you need to build up all of the major muscle groups that interact in and around your back and neck. By supporting and strengthening them, your back will be able to withstand any minor trauma, causing them to relieve any unnecessary pressure around the spine and preventing unnecessarily spasms. Make your muscles harmoniously strong and you will be a much happier person with good posture and a strong back. For this reason, these muscles should be your top priority. This, by the way, is now called "core conditioning" and should be your primary emphasis in your resistance program.

Next, work on your legs because the muscles are larger and will burn up many more calories per hour helping you to lose weight more rapidly. Also, your "wheels" are important for many reasons including; lifting or moving large objects, like your mother-in-law. Safety could also become an issue because of nature's fight or flight principle. Suppose a gunman comes up to you demanding all your money. He's not going to believe you when you tell him that you just spent it all foolishly on some attractive person of the opposite sex you were attempting to pick up in that bowling alley you just left, so you projectile vomit all over him and run away. Since, in that situation, you don't have time to hail a cab, your legs are vital to your well-being. If you haven't run since Lenny Bruce was popular, you could be in deep trouble. Running away could cause all of your muscles to tear at once, leaving you shriveling on the ground like a bowl of Jell-o. Seriously, your legs are more important than your arms, so work them out more. When lifting your grandkids, large packages, pushing, pulling, etc., you should use your legs more than your back or arms. They are larger and more effective for these activities. Plus, most leg exercises involve your arms anyway, so they too will get the benefit of your other exercises.

The arms, especially for men, are the vanity part of this. Yes, vanity is important. Remember, you're doing this for you, so give yourself a little bonus and get some Arnold Schwarzenegger definition in your twigs if you like. The arms need to be strong too, but they will get their own workout from the other things that you do, so no need to worry much about them otherwise.

RULES OF ENGAGEMENT

We need some rules for resistance training, though. Number 1: Never train after drinking a quart of Jim Beam. Number 2: If you do, make sure a commode is nearby. And, number 3: Don't pass out with more than fifty pounds of weights resting on your chest! That might be counterproductive to your plan. Number 4 . . .

Don't just walk in the gym and begin lifting. Also, don't assume that the way you lifted in your previous life was correct. That may be why you quit in the first place. Follow the "Top Ten Rules of Resistance Training" for a healthier and more productive program. (See next page.)

Top ten rules of resistance training;

1. **Warm up, warm down — at least five minutes in the beginning and ten minutes at the end of a session.** Adjust it according to the specific circumstances and ignore any recent study that seems to question the need to stretch.
2. **Slow and steady, steady and slow — take your time and do the exercises the way they were intended.** Learn the proper way to do the specific exercise or machine. There is no race here, and you could very easily hurt yourself. You also may not get the benefit of the exercise by rushing. Generally speaking, the slower you go, the more benefit you will get.
3. **In with the good, out with the bad.** Inhale deeply through your nose and exhale slowly through your mouth in cadence with the particular exercise. Very important!
4. **Set realistic goals.** Strongman competition is not part of the plan. Start out with light weights and work your way up slowly, making sure you're getting between twenty to thirty reps on each set, two sets total.
5. **Variety is the spice of life.** Mix it up and rotate different exercises into your routine for slightly different muscles on a regular basis. You'll continue your newfound passion longer while working out different muscles at the same time, which should also help your overall coordination. Switch to a slightly different exercise for each muscle group (there are plenty to choose from) every three to four months. Your muscles need this variety. Very important, also.
6. **Don't lift over your head.** No military presses especially if you have neck problems. You're just asking for trouble by compressing your vertebrae.
7. **All lifting must be next to your body.** Do not lift weights, babies, groceries, tools, sod, TVs or anything away from your body. Keep them as close as possible to avoid back problems. This could be your most important rule. If you need to lift a large dumbbell, stand next to it, straighten your back, suck in your shrinking gut, begin lifting with your legs, and go slowly.
8. **Make progress.** Begin your program slowly and don't rush to

reach your goals. Remember that you have the rest of your life to get there. On the other hand, making continuing progress is important. As a goal, try to increase your repetition or weight on at least one of your exercises a week.

9. **Quantity, not quantity . . .** Huh? More reps, less weight. The number of repetitions done of each exercise is much more important at this stage of your life than the amount of weight that you are lifting. Reps will build long-term strength or stamina, more weight will put on bulk and the only bulk we want to see is in the produce section of our grocery store. We want to be strong and full of energy all day long, not looking like we're on steroids. Do twenty to thirty reps of each exercise, and do at least two sets of each. This means that you'll probably be using less weight than you thought you would. That's okay. There is always going to be someone in the gym that can lift more than you, so get over the ego thing! You probably need to do at least ten to fifteen different types of exercises to hit all the muscle groups necessary. This should take an hour or two to complete depending on your routine. This point is very important. Decrease the amount of weight you are lifting presently and increase the number of repetitions done to build up your energy reservoirs.
10. **What's up, Doc?** Check with your doctor first to make sure you're not going to do something you'll regret later. (Famous last words!) Your levels of bone loss, arthritic buildup, condition of your heart and lungs, and other factors may determine the level and types of exercises that you can and should do. Your doctor should be able to give you some basic guidelines to follow if you have some physical problems. Use your common sense. Guess we should have put this tip first . . .

If you need help starting a program, there are many different avenues to follow. You can hire a physical trainer to set up a program, buy a video, read a book or magazine, ask someone you know experienced in this area to help or even look for a program already on television. Just make sure that the program is varied and hits all of the muscle groups that we have discussed earlier.

Aerobic exercises

Now that you have a program involving two to three times weekly of resistance type of exercises, you need to do some aerobic activities to build your hearts, lungs, push the blood through your system, blow out your pipes, and burn up some extra calories. If you were to power walk for an hour daily or run three to four miles five days a week, no one would argue that you'd be in great shape. That should be your goal: to be in great aerobic shape with lean, strong and supportive muscles. It can be accomplished in as few as three to four days a week if doing a strenuous enough of an activity; let's say running or climbing stairs. However, walking on a treadmill or walking outside for only twenty to thirty minutes a day will require additional time and effort. You will have to be the judge of how many days weekly are needed to accomplish your goal depending upon the particular type of activities you are doing. Again, it is important to vary your activities for coordination and boredom purposes, but this isn't necessary every time you exercise. You may want to walk four days and run one. Or climb stairs twice and walk three times. Mix it up, but get it done regardless. You may devise a scoring type of a system to motivate you, if you wish. How you keep track of your exercises is also entirely up to you. **There are going to be times when you won't be able to get a full week of workouts done, which is okay, but remember that you are fooling no one but yourself if you slack off. There is no one to make sure that it gets done, no one to stand over you and no one to remind you except you alone. You will see results either way.** If you choose not to exercise, then you will resemble that partially digested burrito we talked about earlier, but whatever you do will be entirely within your control. That's exactly the way it should be.

Consider anything you do that raises your heartbeat for an extended period of time aerobic exercise. Whether it's jogging, power-walking, riding a bike, swimming, mowing, playing tennis, roller-blading, dancing or stepping, it doesn't matter. As long as you are conscious about keeping the activity level up, you'll get the desired effect. Accomplish that several times a week and you'll lose weight, feel better, get healthier and have to buy a whole new set of clothing. Maybe it is expensive to exercise, depending on your taste in clothing!

Balancing Act

One other type of exercising that we haven't discussed involves maintaining your balance throughout your life. Not your balance in life, but the type involving your inner ear, vision, nerves and muscles. **This may not be important when you are fifty, but rest assured that it will be when you reach seventy.** Many, many debilitating accidents occur when an elderly person slips and falls. Whether it be on dry pavement or a slippery sheet of ice, the end result can be the same. You get hurt. You start losing your sense of balance in your mid-twenties, which may explain some drunken stupors of the past. So work on your balance daily.

Try this. Stand on one leg and see how long you can hold it. Don't take this lightly because you probably can't last more than twenty to thirty seconds. Anything that you can devise to challenge your balance will probably be good exercise also, so it can't hurt to spend a few minutes daily on this little aspect of your health. Stand on a balance-board, jump rope, use a stair-climbing machine without resting your hands on the rails and if you have the guts, attempt to use your kid's skateboard. Anything that you can do to challenge your sense of balance will help. It may not seem important now . . .

In summary

Routine exercising needs to be a part of your daily regimen for the rest of your life. You will live longer, be healthier, have more energy and maintain a better attitude. Many forms of cancer will pass you by, as will most colds, viruses, and other immune problems. The onset of arthritis and the aches and pains associated with this crippling disorder will be minimized, and if you eat sensibly you will avoid diabetes. Yes, it takes a lot of work, but as you can see, the effort is well worth it. No health program would be complete without making exercise a crucial part of it. If you're just beginning, give it at least a full two-month trial period. By the time you have exercised for sixty days, the inconvenience and start up aches and pains should be a thing of the past. Like everything else concerning your body (and life in general), momentum is a very difficult thing to get past, and the direction you were probably headed in will be hard to change. Little by little you will see progress and the results. Keep with it and see you at the gym!

"The way to get to the top is to get off your bottom."
–Anonymous

Step 4:

Garbage In . . . Garbage Out

And, "You are what you eat." Two rather old clichés, but they are both as true as they have ever been. While the title implies computer-related jargon, it's very relevant with regards to the fuel you supply your body. In fact, let's throw in one more, "An apple a day keeps the doctor away." Also based on generations of wisdom.

It's imperative at this juncture to fully understand that the quality of the fuel that you put into your system is directly related to the amount and quality of the energy released into and by your body *and* the length of time you will spend on this planet. Put fresh fruits and vegetables, whole grain products and other foods with **high nutritional value** into your stomach and you will maximize the productivity of your body while super-charging your immune system Exist on donuts, potato chips, sodas and Twinkies and the results will be the opposite.

You wouldn't intentionally fill your gas tank with inferior gasoline that you know is going to compromise the integrity of your vehicle, so why eat the wrong foods and jeopardize your well-being? Put corrupted gas into your beautiful new car and the results will be immediate. In other words, you'll know right away that you made a mistake. Your car will sputter and spurt pretty quickly. You body, on the other hand, is so efficient that it generally chugs right through any junk that you put into your mouth leading you to press on and add more and more empty calories to your diet. It does a pretty good job of processing the nutritionally challenged food that you give it. It has done this for years . . . no, decades. Your formerly well oiled machine took every beer, donut, cotton candy, sausage roll, french-fry and bacon double cheeseburger and turned them all into fairly efficient energy. Not any more. Your system has finally said, "Enough is enough. I quit. I am not getting paid nearly enough to take all the crap you feed me in order to make you look good. I am on strike . . . talk to my union steward, the colon. He's fed up too, and you don't not want to hear what he has to say!"

The problem here is that the break down of your different internal components like your digestive, respiratory and immune systems is gradual. Of course, that is by design. You probably wouldn't live very long if your body went into a red alert every time you ate ballpark nachos! Imagine the digestive roller coaster you would go on every time you spiked your blood sugar level from consuming some rather worthless junk food. Think of your worst stomachache happening every time you ate the wrong foods. You'd probably be a whole lot more careful of what you put into your system if that happened all the time. Fortunately your body has been too kind to you.

It should make perfect sense to understand the "garbage in . . . garbage out" philosophy, but do you comprehend this enough to really begin regulating your nutritional intake? There is no in-between. You either believe it or you do not. Can you truly minimize the amount of empty calories you consume? You'll notice that we're not talking about eliminating these completely. We are human, after all. Just keep it to a minimum and you'll be a lot better off. Understand that your body has specific needs from the fuel you supply. Call them specifications if you like. For instance, the intake of vitamin C is extremely important to your health, and is a water-based vitamin that helps your immune system fight colds and the flu along with protecting you against cancer and heart disease, while doubling as a great antioxidant. Most everyone knows that they must get enough of this important element through the food they consume, but what about all the other vitamins? They are equally important also. Vitamins A, all the Bs, D, E and K are just as important to different bodily functions as C is to the above-mentioned ones. If you don't get them from the foods you ingest, then where are they going to come from? Supplements are great, but as the name implies, they are in addition to foods and do not replace high quality foods as your source of much needed nutrition. *Vita* is Latin for vital. If you need one, then you must also need the others. Since your body cannot manufacture most vitamins, they must originate from somewhere other than your body, thus the importance of a good diet. **Your life that you wish to lengthen depends upon enough clean "fuel" to get you there and you cannot rely on supplements. They do not have the same absorption rate and quantity of nutrients that fresh foods do.**

How about calcium? Did you know that calcium is the most abundant mineral in your body? It is necessary for maintaining hard bones and teeth, proper nerve and muscle function and is an essential part of the fluid that surrounds all of your cells. Again, its importance is a no-brainer. However, there are also dozens and dozens of other minerals that are imperative to your good health. **In fact, the majority of illnesses and diseases can be traced to mineral deficiencies of some type.** Where do you plan on getting these if you don't get them from the foods that you eat? Minerals, by nature, are non-organic which means that they don't originate from inside your body. They actually originate from the soil and migrate to the plants and animals before being consumed by humans. So you either have to consume buckets of dirt from different parts of the world, or get them from eating proper foods. The problem is, donuts and Ding Dongs don't contain a whole lot of vitamins and minerals. The point being made here is that the majority of the food you consume must be nutritionally dense. They must contain the vital nutrients that your body needs; otherwise eating junk is a waste and detrimental to your wish to live a long and comfortable life

Momentum

Your internal systems work partially on momentum. Think about it. It has taken several years of abuse, beginning in your twenties, for your body to finally wear down and begin to malfunction. Digestive problems, bone and soft tissue aches and pains, diseases and disorders have crept into your life. In the past, your body would adjust what it ingested to get the job done that it was hired to do, which was to make sure that your bodily functions were operating properly. Things like breathing, talking, walking and yelling at your kids. All the important stuff! As forgiving as your system has been, it can only take *so much* abuse before breaking down. **When you finally begin adding better quality fuel to your system on a regular basis, momentum dictates that the changes you see will be slow in making themselves known.** Eventually you will begin to see a change in the way you feel. Therein lies the problem. It may be two weeks, two months or even longer to see the results, however we generally don't have the patience needed in this instant gratification world of ours. The time it takes for change depends on the efficiency your system already has. You have to remain strong. You need to stick with this program and believe that from now on the quality and length of time you have left on this planet totally depends upon the quality of the fuel you supply your body. Your persistence will pay huge dividends, just not in the next twenty-four hours. Read on. Many of the reasons to eat correctly are outlined here. . .

LET'S GET PHILOSOPHICAL . . . TWO ARGUMENTS FOR A BETTER DIET

What's it going to take to convince you that you need to be careful with the foods you shovel down the chute? That fried foods, glazed donuts and candy bars in the long run will do harm to your body and will eventually wreck the quality and longevity of your life. By consuming junk, you are essentially shortening you life and will cause the last remaining years that you have left on this planet to be downright uncomfortable.

There are several ways to look at the reasons to eat properly, but we can break them down to two basic arguments. First, is the spiritual stance. Put it in a religious perspective and ask; "What would God have to say?" We asked her and this is what she said. (Was there any doubt that God is a woman?) If you believe in God and that God put us here, supplying everything that we need, then ask yourself these questions. Do you think she'd design us with diabetes, heart disease, Alzheimer's or cancer as a part of her design? How about AIDS and pulmonary emphysema? Of course not. It should be obvious that she provided us with *everything* we would need to take proper care of ourselves. Didn't God put onto this earth: fruits, vegetables and other plants to nourish us? God also gave us intelligence (that was her first mistake!) to use and create ways to better ourselves physically and spiritually so that we could build huge churches and pour money into her Swiss bank account. Everything from farming techniques to modern medicine can be attributed to her creation. However, cotton candy was not in her plan. Nor was intelligence that was gifted to us intended to find shortcuts around the common sense systems she left in place for us to use and better ourselves. Bleached flour, white sugar and fried foods weren't a part of the equation.

The foods provided for our use were intended to be eaten whole and raw, not cooked, bleached and processed. Our earth, while protecting us from most of the sun's harmful rays, has been endowed with all the wonderful things we need to take good care of ourselves. All the fruits, vegetables, plant substances, nuts and beans, and of course good pure water have been left here for us to use and manage wisely. Many times it appears that we are not doing such a good job. We have the intelligence to raise livestock to be used for a good source of protein and other nutrients: we then pump them full of antibiotics and hormones. Water has also been provided to cleanse ourselves, nurture our crops and as a medium for our jet-skis. If you have a strong religious upbringing then it's easy to understand this particular reason to take care of yourself by fueling your system only with what was provided for you, and to properly use your God-given intelligence to manage the resources left here by our Creator. It's all here. All the varied anti-oxidants and other crime-fighting nutrients found in all of our naturally occurring foods were put here for a purpose. Use them.

The other side of this coin is the evolution (or survival of the fittest) theory; they are pretty much the same thing. Man began as amoebae (some of us are still there), turned into fish, the fish grew legs and we crawled onto land, probably as turtles. Turtles then turned into monkeys, got better looking and eventually evolved into Mr. Neanderthal (some of us are still there also!). (Note; I may have skipped a couple of steps in the evolutionary process, so please forgive me.) Now Mr. Neanderthal's evolution to modern man took several million years to accomplish. Think about that. Several million years is as long a time as being put on hold by your phone company. The hundreds of thousands of generations have had plenty of time for adaptation and change. In fact, present day man has only been here a fraction of that time.

Survival of the fittest meant that any weaknesses in prehistoric man's system would be culled out and he wouldn't survive to the next set of generations. **Today's man eventually arose because his system was able to make the highest and best use of the vegetation around him, and because of his ability to change with his environment.** It nourished him, helped him grow, made him smarter and kept him going on through time. Internally, his genetic mechanism fine-tuned itself, perfecting and changing its functioning parts and in effect building fail-safe systems to protect him from negative outside influences. Any weakness and inefficiencies died with the premature death of the prehistoric being. Proof? Today, scientists have found a ton of "genetic garbage" left on the human gene that has absolutely no purpose now, but was a result of the evolution of man. This evidence helps prove that the changing of man was a result of his environment and his innate ability to adapt. ***Your* body has been fine-tuned over million of years in order to use your environment and surroundings for your benefit and survival.** In other words, consume the fuels that are indigenous to our lands in their natural state provided for us by evolution and design, and your good health will thrive. Over the millions of generations, man has been fine-tuned to use what was provided him to keep his body healthy.

Only the early humans with strong immune systems survived. The others too weak to fight off disease died and did not reproduce. Don't just look at one generation, but look at hundreds of generations to get a better picture of why we are here and what we really need to put into our systems to assure our survival. This is not far-out Zen-Buddha-philosophical wishful gazing. It is pure evolution at work. **The scary thing is that the American diet has changed more in the last 100 years than it did in the last 1000.**

That is not enough time to adjust in evolutionary terms, thus one of the reason that so many diseases are out of control and at epidemic proportions. It is simple evolution at work. If your pancreas is not strong enough to survive the countless blood sugar spiking of our processed foods of today, then you will not survive, whereas someone with a stronger system will. Very simple. Only the strong will survive to the next generation eventually causing the evolutionary laws to come true. Evolution is at work today, culling out weaknesses at a furious rate and attempting to adapt to the extreme change in man's diet. That is why we are seeing so much disease and death. The strong will survive; the weak will not. Which side of this experiment do you want to be on?

In the United States Patent Office you will find patent number 0000001; the very first patent awarded, which was for the invention called the human body. The inventor is identified only as God. The address given is nebulous, the age and sex unmarked. Only a drawing of a stick person can be found. **Patent #0000001 was the first and the greatest invention we will ever see. For the last 30 years or so you have fed it mostly things with very little nutritional value, better known as garbage, yet it still works pretty damn well considering.** You have shoved the following down your throat: alfredo sauce, bacon, cupcakes, diet sodas, éclairs, funnel cakes, gravy, ham, ice cream, jujubes, and so on down the alphabet for years and years. Your body just kept ticking away. It kept processing all that junk pretty well and you got by, until a few short years ago. Now your internal combustion machine, better known as your gut is coughing and spitting and in general not performing well. Now is the time to change that.

A Crock

Although this program is about you taking control of your life, your diet, per se, is not all your fault. Food manufacturers have done a superb job of convincing you to buy their product, that it is good for you, tastes great and of course your purchase increased their bottom line while increasing your waistline. The following is a good example. We'll call it the second biggest hype of the 90s (after the Y2K buildup). It is food labeling that says "FAT FREE, REDUCED FAT, or LOW FAT." The underlying message is that it's okay to eat this particular food, because its good for you and will not make you fat! What a crock!! Actually, the opposite is true. Your body needs fat to exist. Fat is your friend, to a certain extent. **Carbohydrates are the real weight-gaining enemy.** When a food manufacturer reduces the fat content of a product, they usually add carbs in the form of sugar to make sure that it is still filling and tastes good, and that's how your thighs got to be in two different time zones. Close your eyes and imagine this . . . not now! Wait until you read this example, then close them. Okay, you're standing in a field somewhere in a Midwestern farm community, in between a grain silo and a railroad tanker car. The grain silo is completely filled with cane sugar and the rail car is full of the syrup used to produce your favorite cola drink. Now snap a picture of this scene. **The only thing that you will see in that picture containing even a remote amount of fat is . . . you!** The cane sugar and the cola syrup have absolutely no fat in either one of them. What do you think would happen if you tried to consumed the contents of those storage containers? You'd look like the Fat Bastard character in the Mike Myers films, *Austin Powers.* Not an ounce of fat anywhere inside of those two containers. Let's call them "lite" or "fat free." Technically they both qualify. Sodas are fat free. Cereals, breads, candy and many other things can be fat free, but *you* won't be if you consume too much of any of them.

The point is this: The amount of fat needed in your diet probably needs to be reduced, but the real culprits of weight gain are carbohydrates. Carbs are essential and are needed for energy production by your body. They are very easy to convert to sugar (glucose). However, I would be willing to bet that the number of carbohydrate grams that you consume on a daily basis is way too high and needs to be curbed. A lot less carbs consumed will do what they were intended to do and will help you lose excess poundage. The fat-free claim may be true, but the consequence of consuming them will not be favorable.

Carbohydrates

Carbohydrates are your main source of regular fuel. They are found in: breads, grains, fruits, vegetables, sugar of course, and most drinks containing any calories at all. There was another big farce recently, which was on a Coke can that read "fat free". Yeah, 150 calories, all sugar, but it is technically fat free. Pleeeease! Carbs are important, but to lose weight, you must exhaust all the carbs you have consumed before your body can chip away at those love handles. Then and only then will the pounds come off. *Remember, that magic pill? It really does not exist here.* Cut out the excess carbohydrates alone and you'll probably lose weight and feel better at the same time.

There are basically two types of carbohydrates, simple and complex. You need to know the difference and concentrate on the complex ones, because the simple carbs (sugar types) spike your blood sugar levels too quickly and can subject your poor body to punishment worse than being forced to sit through several *Barney* videos. So, what exactly is the harm in consuming too many simple sugars like sodas, candy bars, etc.? Can you spell D.I.A.B.E.T.E.S? Bad stuff . . . You will die faster from diabetes complications than from moving in with your in-laws! **Consuming too many simple carbohydrates puts an incredible strain on your pancreas, liver and the remainder of your digestive system.** The constant strain can cause your magnificent system to fail, pure and simple. Your carburetor will go kaput. Your fuel filter will explode and your gas tank will rot away! Diabetes is not a pleasant disease. Loss of limbs is not unusual; heart attacks are very common, and blindness can follow. Diabetes also requires a regime that, once you have been unfortunate enough to contract this horrible disease, is a huge pain in the butt to follow. Diabetes is a result of putting too much of a strain on your digestive system, especially your pancreas, and of adding too much weight on your body's frame through overeating. The biggest culprits are the simple carbohydrate (sugar), generally not the fat you consume. The simple sugars get into your blood way too quickly, spiking your blood sugar level too high, too fast, forcing your pancreas to work overtime pumping out insulin that regulates the amount of sugar absorbed into your body. The simple truth is that eventually your pancreas breaks down and quits producing the needed insulin. You now have diabetes. If not treated, you will die a fairly quick and painful death. Once your pancreas breaks down, it cannot be fixed. You're stuck with this debilitating disease for the rest of your shortened life. **The way to preserve your pancreas and even more important liver is to give it only the complex carbs and allow your organs to work at their own pace.** Rev up your car's engine too many times and it will blow. The difference is that you can always fix your car . . . rev your body's engine too much and it will simply go on a permanent strike.

Your (soon to be) formerly abused body really only needs the complex carbs to run smoothly. They are broken down slower and steadier, so as not to spike Mr. Blood Sugar Level and make him mad. They are simply much better for you. Examples of complex carbohydrates are; whole grains and whole grain products, most vegetables, some fruits, legumes (beans), and Cheeze Whiz. (Just kidding on that last one.) Concentrate on these type of carbs and you will be much better off. The harder it is to turn a carbohydrate into useable sugar, the better it is for your system. In this case, slower is better. Cotton candy goes immediately into your blood while whole grain breads take a while, thus are better for you. Rice can be used as a good example. Undercook it to the point that it is chewy and your digestive system will have a harder time breaking it down, thus it goes into your blood supply very slow. Overcook it and it will enter your blood very quickly, spiking the blood sugar level. This is another reason to eat your plant-based foods as raw as is possible.

Fat

Fats need to be an essential part of your diet because of their use in cell division and maintenance. It's their misuse and overuse that gets you in trouble. Fats are a specific chain of carbon atoms with hydrogen atoms attached. They can be classified by whether all of the available carbon atoms are occupied (saturated) with hydrogen atoms or not.

The carbon atoms of the saturated fats are completely occupied with hydrogen atoms. Most all saturated fats, which are solid at room temperature, are found in beef, lamb, whole milk products like butter and cream, un-skinned chicken and many processed foods made from palm and coconut oils. Stay away from these. They contain, and will help contribute to, high levels of cholesterol in your body.

Margarine, solid vegetable shortening and many other foods made from "partially hydrogenated oils" are unnatural sources of saturated fats and may actually be worse on your system than the previously mentioned fats. These products are made from vegetable oils that have been artificially saturated with hydrogen to make them at least semi-solid at room temperature. Hydrogen is "forced" into each and every molecule. That fact, by itself, should be enough to raise a red flag. Their danger lies in the fact that they are chemically unstable allowing them to react with oxygen, which can result in DNA and cell membrane damage. Quite simply, this can lead to degenerative changes in your body's tissue, abnormal inflammation and even cancer. Also, when these partially hydrogenated oils are treated with solvents or heated, their atoms can deform into an unnatural or jointed shape commonly known as trans-fatty acids. **Trans-fatty acids can do damage to your immune system because their toxicity hinders your system's battle against disease and other maladies that it faces daily. The fact that they are unnatural and rarely found in nature should be enough reason to stay away from these.** These are bad news and need to be eliminated from your diet or you'll be sabotaging your effort to improve your health. You're better off eating chicken fat than trans-fat.

The following is a list of products that you might not have realized contain partially hydrogenated oil: most candies, Ritz Bits and Ritz crackers, Triscuits and Wheat Thins, Honey Graham Crackers, Saltine crackers, most cookies and crackers, margarine, shortening, tortilla chips, some potato chips, cakes, brownies, packaged donuts, fried foods, cream type dressings, store bought biscuits, energy bars (that's surprising), and the list of other like products goes on. Bummer, huh! Read the labels!!! Take most of these products out of your daily diet and you'll feel better and losing weight will be easier.

If you consume too high of a percentage of saturated fats your liver will make too much LDL, (the bad cholesterol) which your body will be unable to use or remove through proper circulation. The result can be an accumulation of this plaque-type substance on your arterial walls (arteriosclerosis), heart disease in general and any other malady caused or aided by blood flow restriction.

Much better for you than saturated fats, polyunsaturated fats are found in corn, sesame, sunflower, safflower and soy oils. These have several carbon atoms unspoken for and are okay for you unless they have been converted into the partially hydrogenated variety. Read the ingredient label on the product before putting it into your shopping cart.

Monounsaturated oils such as olive, peanut, canola and even avocado seem to be the top choice among the fats to choose from with olive being the best by far. Olive oil actually helps reduce the level of the bad cholesterol, and its fatty acid, called oleic acid, seems to be accepted easier into your body. The olive tree is very hardy and disease free. The oil from its fruit has been used for thousands of years and the countries that use predominately olive oil have a lower incident of heart disease. The extra-virgin type, which is preferred, means that they sacrifice a virgin in the processing of the oil, which is then approved by the god of oil. It's then extracted by cold pressing and isn't made with solvents or excessive heat. The other monounsaturated fats listed above do not, in general, have that distinction. Olive oil (not Popeye's girlfriend) is by far your best choice to use in the kitchen. This is another one of those common sense items. Use olive oil whenever possible. You can even use it in the bedroom, but you won't get quite the same results.

There is also one other fat to discuss and it is called Omega-3 fatty acids. Omega-3s are highly unsaturated fatty acids that also have beneficial characteristics which include: lowering cholesterol, protecting against cancer, reducing negative inflammatory changes to your body and protecting it against abnormal blood clotting and degeneration at the cellular level in general. It is a good idea to make this a part of your daily regime either through supplements containing flax seed oil or ground up seeds, fish oils, or by eating cold water fish. These include sardines, salmon, herring, tuna, etc. Flax seed is extremely inexpensive and can be ground up to use in salads, cereal or soups. You must buy it fresh though and don't grind it until needed. It tends to spoil quickly. Find a convenient source of omega-3 fatty acids and include them in your diet. Omega-3 and omega-6 fatty acids usually come together and are both needed to get the results that you are searching for.

A general rule as far as fats are concerned is as follows:

Limit your fat intake to about 20–25% of your normal daily

calorie consumption and of those fats avoid the saturated kind whenever possible. Stay away from most processed foods for they will probably contain partially hydrogenated oils and too much fat. Concentrate on poly and monounsaturated oils (olive) and add in some Omega-3 fats as much as you can.

PROTEINS

Repairs, growth and development of new tissues require the consumption of a protein source. A deficiency in protein can cause major damage to your body's healing process. Thankfully, most Americans do not have that problem. In fact, many times, we get too much.

Proteins are amino acids, many of which are essential to proper body function. Some cannot be manufactured by your body meaning that they must be consumed in your diet. Sources of protein are: meats, dairy products, poultry, fish, beans and many vegetables. Getting your quota of protein is not generally the problem. Consuming protein without a large amount of fat catching a ride along is the tricky part. **Stick to only lean cuts of meat and poultry, use reduced-fat dairy products, search for low-fat cheeses and yogurts and try and get more of your protein from vegetable and bean sources rather than from animals.** Soy products are also fantastic.

Note: beans are a great source of protein without the negative characteristics of meats.

If you are a vegetarian, make sure that you consume enough vegetable protein and supplement your diet with all of the B vitamins since you probably don't get enough of either.

Generally speaking, carbohydrates, fats and proteins are the tools used by your body to regulate the millions and millions of chemical reactions that go on inside of your body each and every day. Keep these in balance, of good quality and from fresh sources and your body will be forever grateful.

LITTLE CRITTERS

There is one aspect of your digestive system that I'm sure you have never thought about. It's an extremely important facet of digestion that most people never consider, but you will now. To demonstrate, let's do an experiment. Stand inside of your coat closet and close the door. Look around and count the number of living things that are with you. If you tallied less than several trillion living organisms, you were wrong. Besides all of the mites and other creatures in the carpeting and in the materials making up your jackets and coats, there are millions and millions of microorganisms on your skin, in your scalp and hair. . . Forget about those nasty little varmints. The ones that we're concerned with are the trillions of microorganisms that should be living in your digestive system. Isn't that a comforting thought?

Don't worry, though. The vast majority of these cute little guys that are living comfortably inside of you are extremely beneficial and are supposed to be there. In a healthy intestinal tract there are over 500 different species of little bacteria residing there and they make up approximately two to three pounds of your body's weight. Thank God they are on your side! They are there for several reasons including: assisting in the digestive process, cleaning up your intestinal tracts by feeding on the waste, fungi, unwanted yeast, harmful bacteria and other poisons while also aiding your body in producing many essential things such as vitamins, proteins and hormones. They compete for food with the harmful microbes that are there to do you harm, and will indirectly starve them off while completing their other functions, like aiding in the absorption of calcium, magnesium and zinc, the enhancement of your immune system and the formation of many crucial substances such as lactic acid, hydrogen peroxide and antioxidants. Without them, your entire system would be (or already is) in the proverbial "world of hurt." If you're not carrying around those couple of pounds of beneficial bacteria in your intestines, your entire system becomes as inefficient as our federal government. It's akin to not having any method of cleaning out your automobile's fuel system. If not cleaned our regularly, (today's gasoline has cleaning agents built in) your car would become very sluggish and wouldn't run well in general. If never treated, that inaction would greatly shorten the life of your motorized vehicle. Not having these special guys homesteading in your intestines will lead to many problems and maladies, some very serious, unless you don't consider death as being serious.

Knowing about these beneficial organisms and keeping them in plentiful abundance is as important as any information you can learn to improve your health!

Years and years of antibiotic misuse, diseases, poor dietary habits, alcohol use, drinking chlorinated water, stress and other abuses to your body have all contributed to the annihilation of the bacterial colonies that are supposed to be residing in your intestinal tract. How important is this?

The following is a list of some of the ailments and problems associated with having inadequate levels of beneficial organisms in your tummy:

- chronic fatigue and anemia,
- allergies,
- frequent diarrhea,
- bladder infections,
- vitamin B deficiencies,
- increased PMS symptoms,
- hormonal imbalances,
- immune system failures,
- constipation and gas,
- high cholesterol,
- candida infections,
- chronic bad breath.

Read this again. It should be obvious that good health is difficult to achieve without having your little buddies around. Having beneficial bacteria in your system is similar to turbo-charging your car. It is the same basic car, but with a lot more power (energy), and it will last a lot longer.

An American Epidemic

Most Americans have done as complete and thorough a job of annihilating their beneficial bacteria friends residing in their intestines as our ancestors did in wiping out the vast majority of the Native American Indian population residing in the New World. One example is antibiotic misuse. Every time that you have taken antibiotics, on top of the bugs you were ***trying*** to rid yourself of, you were virtually wiping out your entire colony of *beneficial* bacteria that, until now, was not replenished. The overuse of antibiotics in America has done more to harm our health than grunge music and *The Osbornes.* **Antibiotics are like Napalm. They don't know the difference between the bad and beneficial bacteria. They wipe out most all of the bacteria, allowing a few remaining harmful bacteria to get a foothold in your digestive system.** That's when the trouble begins. What you have just accomplished by this example is to begin to breed a super strain of bacteria. Only the strong ones survived the antibiotics. Does this sound familiar? As a result, we now have antibiotic-resistant super-bacteria that are virtually untreatable and many times fatal. By wiping out your beneficial intestinal bacteria, you also lose most of your ability to fight off illnesses of many kinds. There is a certain balance between the beneficial and harmful bacteria in your body. It's designed to be like the Cold War. The good guys keep the bad guys in check, which, in turn, keep you healthy. **Prescribing antibiotics for most colds and the flu, which are caused by viruses and not bacteria, does absolutely no good in fighting that type of ailment. Get you and your family off of antibiotics now and start rebuilding your little health warriors.** As mentioned above, there are already some nasty antibiotic resistant bacteria out there for which medical science has no cure for. In fact, there are some specialized ones residing inside of hospitals just waiting for you to visit. **The over-prescribing of antibiotics is an example of how we now have ailments and**

diseases caused by the people and industry charged with protecting our health. And you want to entrust your entire health maintenance to the medical profession? This, by itself should make you think a little.

There are two different types of microorganisms that need to be renting condos inside of your intestines. The more familiar ones mentioned above can be ingested by eating soured products such as: cultured yogurt, cottage cheese, buttermilk, sour kraut, whey and your mother-in-law's cooking. This category within your diet should be satisfied a few times a week, which should be rather easy to do. A good yogurt product can take care of most of this requirement and makes a great meal when other fruits and cereals are added to the mix. Eat any of these several times weekly. They contain some acidophilus and other lactobacillus necessary for a healthy intestinal environment. It's also a good idea to give your yogurt a boost by adding a quarter teaspoon of acidophilus (found at any health food store) to each serving. The probiotic enzymes that you can also purchase from GNC or a health food store are also a good idea. They contain some of the other strains of bacteria, giving you a well rounded variety of residents in your gut. Your colon will thank you . . .

Eat dirt

The second type is rather obscure and most people don't even know they exist. These are soil-based microorganisms that we'll call SBOs. Finding SBOs never used to be problem when we were primarily a farming country, and as far back as our cave days. Every time humans would eat something straight out of the ground or directly from a farm, they ingested some SBOs which would take up residence in your intestines and provide you with the benefits that they were meant to provide. Another way of looking at this is that they actually ate a little dirt. Not much, but enough to get a colony of SBOs started. Could that be why little kids eat dirt? Maybe they are supposed to! Eating just a microscopic bit of the right soil will give you the benefit of these very beneficial microorganisms. Today, our food sources are overfarmed, over-processed, sprayed, irradiated and cooked to death resulting in a rather sterile product devoid of some of the things that you never realized that you needed. Without getting into a lot of details about SBOs, they do benefit you in the following ways similar to the first type of microorganisms mentioned. They eliminate accumulated putrefaction in your intestinal walls, where harmful organisms can get their start. They will continue to break down foods to their most basic elements allowing for total and complete absorption by your body also negating the need for excess food to accomplish that. SBOs will help stimulate your immune system and are also very aggressive against molds, yeast, fungi and viruses. In addition, they help metabolize proteins for your cells and rid the cells of toxic waste. SBOs have done miraculous things for people with a variety of diseases and ailments and should be taken as a part of your diet for at least a short period of time until they get a chance to take hold and begin their work inside of your digestive system. Antibiotics also kill these friendly little guys. It would help you to replenish these at least once. (SBOs may be difficult to find in conventional health food stores, but you can find SBOs through a company called Life Science Products at 435-628-4111.) Eating a lot of raw organic produce may help you get SBOs too, but don't count on it.

There *will* be times in the future that you will need to take antibiotics. These include: actual bacterial infections, surgery, wounds, kissing your Aunt Ethel, etc. When you are finished, take special steps to replenish your little friends to keep your system running "on all eight cylinders." Having a healthy population of intestinal bacteria cannot be overemphasized. They are absolutely crucial to you health and well being. If you have wiped out their presence by the previously mentioned habits and maladies, take all the steps you can to replenish them immediately.

DIETS

We Americans are obsessed with weight loss and dieting, so much so that literally billions of dollars are spent annually in the diet industry. Yet we are still fat, obese, overweight, tubby, or anything else you wish to call it. The truth is that most diets are just gimmicks and just don't work for a variety of reasons.

There are hundreds of different diets available today. There is the Atkin's Diet that encourages you to eat mostly fat and cut carbs almost completely out of your regime. This is a good program if you are extremely overweight since your obesity is a bigger problem than not eating fruits and vegetables, at least for a while. Once you have the weight under control, you're better off with a more balanced diet.

How about the grapefruit diet? This plan encourages you to eat a grapefruit at each meal, which is fine since grapefruit is a very good antioxidant. However, if that keeps you from eating other fruits and vegetables, then it's probably not a good idea. Plus grapefruits don't increase your metabolism as the diet says, and they can actually increase the potency of medications you may be taking by speeding the rate of absorption into your system. This is not a good diet.

There is actually a diet based upon your specific blood type. I don't think so . . .

The Zone Diet is a more balanced plan that forces you to consume 40% of your calories from carbohydrates, 30 from fat and 30 from protein. Not bad, but probably too much protein and fat.

Dr. Bob Arnot's Revolutionary Weight Control Program wants you to eat mostly carbohydrates, which raises the level of serotonin released into your system supposedly curbing your hunger. Again, this is not balanced enough. Carbohydrates are important, but Americans continually stuff their faces with all sorts of carbs and it has lead only to more eating, not less.

The Ornish Diet restricts the intake of fat to about 10% which is a good idea but may be difficult to stick to. The Sugar

Busters plan calls for the elimination of almost all sugars including simple sugars (soft drinks, sweets, etc.) and complex carbohydrates (rice, beans, breads, etc.). Getting rid of the simple sugars is a great idea. Quitting the complex carbs is not. Long grain rice, beans, whole grain wheat, vegetables and fruits fall into this category and are extremely important to good health.

The Weight Watchers plan is seems to be the best diet plan of all the offerings today because it is based in portion control, but still uses "point counting" which is just another gimmick to get you to stop eating too much of the wrong foods. There are so many diet plans out there, we could go on for days analyzing them, but won't.

You'll notice medical doctors author the vast majority of diet plans that don't work. That's the same doctor with the same training that you want to trust your life to, yet they can't even seem to agree on what is best for you to eat . . . just something to think about.

My Diet Plan

You only need one diet plan and that is mine. It is accordingly called **My Diet Plan.com.** (I just added the "dot-com" part) I'd like to announce my brand new, revolutionary, cutting edge, high tech, and exciting diet discovery. It's so profound that it will take your breath away. It's also extremely effective because it is very simple. You cannot find this anywhere else but here. It took volumes of research and years to perfect. It can be used from now until the day that you die, which will be a lot longer than otherwise since you purchased this book. The pounds will just pour off of you in a very short period of time, and it's also free-my gift to you. (Just send $29.95 to cover shipping.) Neighbors will whistle, friends will start calling, you'll get that promotion you've wanted, and your luck will change dramatically. The science is sound, the rational solid, the technique simple. Hundreds of people have lost thousands of pounds on this incredible diet and so will you.

Okay, are you ready to be impressed? Are you seated? Here it goes . . . My New Diet Plan in a nutshell is as follows:

Consume less calories that you use, on a daily basis.

Or stated differently:

Burn off more calories that you take in every day.

Wow! Pretty exciting isn't it? You don't need to eat twelve grapefruit a day. There is nothing special to eat for your specific blood type. Don't eat all proteins or carbohydrates. Don't run in place for thirty minutes before dining and you don't have to buy food from any special place. Eat balanced meals using the nutritionally sound principles outlined here and simply use more calories daily than you eat and you will lose weight. If you burn off 2500 calories a day and consume only 2000, then you will lose about a pound a week. Pretty simple stuff since you are now going to be smart about what you shovel down your throat. You are also now going to read labels, cut out sweet sodas, eat a variety of fruits, vegetables and whole grains. You're going to start exercising on a regular basis for the rest of your life, and you're going to watch your portion sizes, cutting out the fatty dressings, toppings and desserts. You're just going to be food smart while micro-managing your digestive system, and it is going to work!

Actually, offering you a "diet plan" is an insult to your intelligence. You don't need a specific point-counting, grapefruit concentrate, 60/30/10, journal-keeping gimmicky diet. Just eat the right foods, add exercise to your regime and the weight will come off. This is not rocket science. It's nothing more than common sense. Don't eat junk. From now on, less is more when it comes to your food intake. **In fact, recent studies have shown that people that have the *best* success losing weight and keeping it off, do not follow any specific diet plan at all!** Don't get sucked into another gimmick.

TEN WEIGHT-LOSS GUIDELINES

To help you out, all you need are some guidelines and controls. The following are ten steps that will help you monitor what goes past those teeth of yours. You still have your teeth, don't you? Good. This helpful list combined with the ten guidelines on eating that you'll read about next is all you need to know to help lose poundage and maintain your ideal weight.

1. **Drink a big glass of water 30 minutes before each meal.** You need eight glasses daily anyway, and a glass a half hour before a meal will help fill you up. (Drink it too close to the meal may interfere with your digestive enzymes.)
2. **Always leave something on your plate.** After the spy plane incident with the Chinese, I no longer care if there are "people starving in China" as our parents continually told us as children. Always leave some of the high calorie foods like meats, breads, loaded baked potatoes, etc. on your plate when you are finished, especially when dining out. You do not need to "get your money's worth" out of a restaurant meal. Let the busboys feast on what you leave behind!
3. **Eat out less often.** Take a look around your typical restaurant. There are usually a higher than average percentage of heavy people dining. There would be a reason for that. Excessively dining out will put excessive weight on. If you have no choice because of work and or travel, then be smart. A restaurant can be your friend if you work at it. You can order just what you need and nothing else. You can get all the servings of vegetables and fruits that you need without the waste you normally have at home. The proper amount of protein is readily available, and you don't have to worry about spoilage or out of date things growing in your fridge! If it's just for pleasure, save some money and have more healthy meals at home.
4. **Read food labels!!!** Very important. Before you decide to have a package of crackers instead of a healthier alternative, see how

many grams of fat and carbohydrates are in the total number of servings you are about ready to eat. Also check for partially hydrogenated vegetable oils. I'll bet that trans-fatty acid is part of the ingredients. If so, make a wiser choice. How many calories are you going to eat? Read, read and read some more.

5. **Don't eat after a certain time.** Begin at, lets say 8:00 PM and don't eat after that time for a week, then 7:45 PM the next week and so on until you're going three to four hours without eating before bed. That will effectively shrink your tummy making you less hungry in the long run. It will also give your digestive system a break.
6. **Fill up on volume foods that don't have high calorie counts.** Broth soups (not creamed), vegetable juices, water, raw vegetables, etc. The reason should be obvious. They will make you feel full.
7. **Grazing.** Eat smaller meals, maybe five times a day instead of the usual three. Your stomach will shrink and your metabolism will be higher because your digestive system will be busier, longer. Be careful not to consume more calories than you would otherwise. Grazing is considered better for you because of putting less strain on your entire digestive process in general. Just make sure that you go some fairly long periods without eating so as to give your digestive system a break. Eating five or six meals a day burns more calories than just two or three, assuming the same calorie intake.
8. **Chew gum immediately before and after eating.** Before to stimulate saliva production and after to keep the process going. While we're on the subject of chewing, be sure and chew your food longer than you probably do now. It's easier on your stomach and will make you feel full quicker.
9. **Brush your teeth often.** You won't want to eat if you just brushed your teeth. Hungry? Go brush your teeth. It also fights acid reflux.

10. **Think thin.** Your mind is the most powerful thing that you own, so use it. Tell yourself that you are going to lose weight, get thin, lose those inches and buy those new clothes after taking off the weight. Of course the best trick is to take your clothes off and stand in front of a mirror. That should be all the encouragement that you need to convince yourself to get on the bandwagon and stop stuffing yourself. Just make sure that mirror is located in the privacy of your home and not in public!

Ten General Food Guidelines

A proper diet does not need to be complicated to work. By eating healthy you will lose weight and increase the health of your entire system at the same time. If you can remember these ten easy rules concerning the food that you consume you'll have a pretty good handle on providing a complete and healthy source of fuel for your ever-demanding system. By keeping the rules simple and less complicated it becomes easier to accomplish your dietary goals.

1. **Don't discriminate.** It is against the law to discriminate against people of color, race, and musical preferences. The same should be true of the foods that you eat. Keep it colorful. **If you eat different colors of foods, and as long as they are fresh and unprocessed, you'll probably be getting most of the minerals, vitamins, fiber and other elements that your system needs to function properly.** Note: Twinkies do not qualify as a colorful food for our discussion here. Carrots, tomatoes, spinach, green beans, kidney beans, broccoli, sweet potatoes, red apples, green apples, red grapes, green grapes, and red onions are just some of the colorful fresh foods that are very potent in life-extending nutrients. These foods contain an incredible amount of phytonutrients that supply life saving antioxidants. Antioxidants are your primary source of disease and cancer fighters. Each different food and each different color introduce unique specialists that fight many different ailments. Thus the need to colorize your diet.

"Man cannot survive on bread alone," so along with the whole grains, add some protein sources, sprinkle in some fat, and eat lots of fruits and vegetables. There is no rule or law that says that you must have meat at every dinner. Fish and poultry are good substitutes for beef. In fact, you can do very well with salads, soy, legumes (beans), and different vegetables without even introducing animal proteins at the dinner table. Again, mix it up. Variety is the key. Broccoli is a great food, but not every night for dinner! Be creative, colorful and keep it interesting. If you introduce different colors at every meal, your diet will benefit tremendously. Remember color every time you go to the grocery store.

2. **Moderation.** National Medal of Science winner and U. C. Berkeley biochemist Bruce Ames **has shown that about half of all the chemicals on this planet, whether natural or synthetic, cause cancer in animals if they are delivered in high enough doses. In other words, an excess of anything is not good for your health.** Steak is a wonderful way to treat yourself occasionally, but you don't need a 42-ounce cut at one sitting, nor do you need to partake in that ritual daily! Order a small one occasionally. A normal portion should be about the size of a deck of cards, probably around six to eight ounces. In fact, that's the normal acceptable portion of most main dishes, whether it's red meat, poultry, pork, fish or pasta. Do you want a piece of chocolate? Again, a small piece once in a while will do you no harm. Have a drink of alcohol, an ice cream cone, an order of nachos, a donut or virtually anything as long as you don't overdo it. If 98% of your diet is healthy, you will not hurt your system with an occasional treat. The treat will be of great help to your moral, curb cravings and will make eating healthy easier to accomplish. Don't eat too much of one type of food product alone, like breads and grains. Don't drink gallons of fruit juices, as they are not a good source of fiber and contain

way too much sugar. Have one glass a day to get a dose of the nutrients. A couple of cola drinks a week won't hurt, but several colas a day will. Besides the sugar, most colas contain phosphoric acid which will leech the calcium out of your bones! Not a good idea at your age. One to two cups of coffee a day can be of benefit. Six cups will not. A glass of wine nightly will give you some good antioxidants and help protect your heart. A bottle a night is obviously counterproductive. If you have a weight problem, then obviously you need to be more careful with your diet, but by moderating everything you put into your system, you'll be much better off. **Moderation allows you to add a variety of needed nutrients to your diet by simply leaving room for other foods while keeping your body from having to cope with excesses of any kind.** This applies to everything from coffee to T-bones and ice cream to pizza. Just remember, the only one you will fool by trying to work and abuse this rule is you. No one else really cares but you.

3. **When less is more.** There are some interesting studies going on that explore the idea of eating less than the supposedly minimum calories needed for maintaining good health. The initial results point toward adding years to your life by subtracting calories from your daily diet. The one key is making sure the calories that you do consume are of good quality and that essential vitamins and minerals are supplemented daily. In other words, if a 2000-calorie a day diet is good for you, then maybe a 1600 daily intake of calories would be better. Part of the theory is that every time you eat, free radicals are released into your system as a natural bi-product of metabolism. Less consumed, less free radicals released. Very interesting research! ***The main point here is not to overeat.*** It's just not good for you. Stuffing yourself literally puts a strain on your system. Your stomach is stretched, your digestive system

goes into overdrive trying to process the excess food, and your heart is forced to pump more blood to your digestive system, taking blood away from your brain (that's why you get sleepy). Your digestive system also needs an occasional break from its job and will only get one when there is nothing available to process. You don't pump more gasoline into your car that it holds because the results are immediate. The same is true in your stomach. Contrary to your motorized vehicle, sometimes it's better to let your tank "run dry." Eat less and live longer. Don't starve yourself! All you need to do if you wish to explore this avenue is to cut down your total caloric intake, wisely.

4. **Read all available food labels!!!** This cannot be emphasized enough. Do not be fooled by the color of the food or the description on the container. **Go directly to the label. Do not buy any food before reading the food content label. You *will* be surprised and dismayed at what you find.** Begin with the ingredients portion first. The most abundant ingredient will be listed first and then in descending order down to the least prevalent one. If you are buying breads, crackers, or other grain items you want the ingredients to begin with "100% whole wheat," "100% whole grain" or some other type of a complete grain. What you'll probably see 98% of the time is going to be "multigrain, wheat flour, enriched wheat blah, blah, blah." It is basically processed white flour. When you read about fiber later on, you'll see what you're missing by eating less than whole grains. You may have to get these necessary bread items at some sort of health foods store. That's okay though because the taste difference and the health benefits are significant and worth the trip. Back on the label, you're also looking for sugar, sucrose, fructose, malted barley, molasses or anything else that adds sugar (simple carbs) into the mix. You will usually see some sugar added, but keeping it to a minimum will help keep your blood sugar level and your weight down. Generally speaking,

the longer the list of ingredients the more chance of there being items you are not going to want to put into your body. There should be little or no saturated fats and preferably some mono-unsaturated fats, if any fats at all. Many times food manufacturers will add a ton of salt to bring out the flavor, so make sure that the sodium level is not sky high, too. If you're concerned about your weight, then you must watch the carbohydrate level in the foods that you consume. A high amount of carbs will kill a good diet in a hurry! As an example, a good breakfast can have over a hundred grams of carbohydrates by itself! A breakfast bar can have 50 by itself. God only knows how many carbs are in a large piece of pizza! Count your carbs as much as you do your calories. If there are ingredients on the label that you cannot even pronounce, then beware. Again, read every label you can. Be an educated food consumer. Once you get used to a better diet, processed foods will taste less appealing anyway.

5. **If it tastes too good to be true, then . . .** it probably is. I don't know of any food that tastes rich, creamy, sweet, full of flavor or is "to die for" that's not fattening or just bad for you. Pizza, chocolate cake, ranch dressing, potato salad, double bacon cheeseburgers, french fries, muffins, pancakes with syrup, garlic bread, fried pies, milk shakes, etc. It is more than likely not in your best interests to make a regular habit of eating these types of foods. Splurge occasionally but remember that moderation is the key. Any one of these items can crush your efforts to cut down on your calorie consumption on a daily basis, so you have to be very careful what you put in your mouth. Note: refer back to the "Fat Boys" section of this book for some hideous examples. The temptations abound! Remember that the devil comes in many shapes, sizes and flavors!
6. **The incredible bulk.** Adding more fiber to your diet is crucial in your quest for optimum health. Whole grain fiber is rich in

vitamins, minerals and antioxidants. Fruit and vegetable fiber along with the fiber found in beans, oats and whole grains also serve several purposes in your digestive system. The soluble type found in beans, soy, oats and fruits assists in lowering levels of cholesterol and insulin in your blood which can reduce your risk of coronary heart disease and diabetes. You can think of it as scrubbing and rinsing away the plaque buildup in your arteries and then flushing it out of your system. Since it dissolves in water and becomes gelatin like in your digestive tract, it also makes you feel full and less likely to overeat.

The insoluble fiber found in vegetables, wheat bran and whole grains is just that. It is unable to be absorbed by your body, so it passes through. On its way out, it absorbs water making your stools softer and bulkier (isn't it amazing all the things that excite us as we age!) and hastens their progress through the large intestine. Let's also not forget constipation and hemorrhoids. The speeding of food through your digestive system keeps you from straining unnecessarily allowing you to read your newspaper comfortably while taking care of business. What happens if your car's muffler becomes clogged or damaged? The correlation is the same as your digestive system. If you fail to keep your intestines scrubbed clean, the ensuing buildup will not only render your system ineffective, it can lead to many life threatening ailments including colon cancer, obesity, diabetes, and diverticular disease (when small sacs balloon out from your colon's wall-very bad). Many, many nutrients are absorbed into your blood stream by passing through the lining in your intestines. If the linings are covered in *you know what,* then the lack of nutrients absorbed into your blood stream opens up the flood gates for many other problems. **In fact it is safe to say that most problems that you can be inflicted with begin as a lack of some sort of nutrient whether it be a vitamin or mineral and thus it can be argued**

that the process starts in your intestines! You have to keep your muffler, chimney and your exhaust system free of the junk that clutters up the walls or you're asking for problems. As in a combustion engine, if the exhaust mechanism is gummed up, the engine will lose much efficiency and its life will most definitely be shortened.

Since our diets are so centered around breads, let's discuss the benefits of whole grain in your diet. Around the turn of the century (actually, the previous one) all of our bread was made from whole grain. White flour wasn't even available until the late 1800s. After white bread grabbed a foothold in the American diet, problems began occurring. Obvious vitamin and mineral deficiencies leading to many diseases was found to be centered around our lack of whole grain consumption. The nutritional output of the American bread was so lacking that in 1943 a federal requirement put back into white processed flour, iron and some B vitamins. Later on folic acid, another B vitamin was also added. Amazing, the organic nutrients were originally stripped out of the product, and then artificially added back. That makes a lot of sense. **Even so, enriched four is not anywhere near the equivalent of whole grain flour.**

It's very easy to see what is lacking when you know what is removed in the milling process. The whole grain's outer covering called the bran contains; vitamin E, zinc, copper, several B vitamins, magnesium, antioxidants and disease fighting agents called phytochemicals, not to mention all the fiber. This all-important bran is removed. The wheat germ, or inner core also contains vitamins and minerals and that too is removed. All that is left is the protein filled starchy substance called the endosperm, which has little to no value. **So when you eat white bread, you are receiving no nutritional benefit, which means that you must get it from some other source causing you to overeat until that requirement is satisfied.** Isn't that the definition of junk food? Substitute whole grain when you can, and eat more vegetables and fruits. Throw in some beans and the increased fiber from all of these will add years to your life and you'll feel better at the same time.

7. **Eat me raw!** The less your food is cooked, the more nutrition is available for you to ingest. Eat your broccoli raw and you get all of the nutrients. Steam it slightly and the benefit is still there. Boil it in water for forty-five minutes and there's not much left in the way of vitamins and minerals. **If you have to cook your fruit or vegetable, then steaming is by far the best method.** If you haven't bought your steamer yet, then add a very small amount of water in the bottom of a pan, add the food, cover and cook for as short of time as possible (maybe five to ten minutes max). ***Don't boil the heck out of your food!*** Look at the water after overcooking. All the nutrients are sent down the kitchen drain! You're wasting most of the value associated with that particular food. All the vitamins, minerals and antioxidants are either destroyed or washed away by incinerating your poor food. **Overcooking foods is one of the biggest tragedies in the American kitchen. Remember that your body requires you to eat a specific food for a particular reason and if you don't fulfill that nutrient then you'll continue eating until your body thinks it has been satisfied.** Eating your fruits and vegetables as close to raw as is possible is your best option for good health. If unavailable, flash frozen is not a bad choice. That type of processing has improved tremendously over the years, locking in more flavor, nutrients and fiber. (By making salads a large part of your diet, you can satisfy this guideline.)
8. **Eat out less often.** A restaurant can be your best friend or your worst enemy. For most people it's the latter. **Restaurants are a fertile breeding ground for obesity.** Sorry, but that's the reality of eating out in today's American restaurants. There are several problems associated with dining out. First, the portion sizes are

huge, sometimes several times the safe or normally suggested amounts. Secondly, to make the food taste ever so good, butter, cream, excess salts and other unhealthy (but wonderful tasting) ingredients are added. The end result is that you can get your entire daily calorie, fat, carbohydrate and/or sodium requirement in one meal! If you eat outside the home often, you can gain enough weight to be assigned your own zip code. So cut down the number of times you dine out monthly and save a ton of money.

Eating out one less time a month can more than pay for a thirty day supply of all the nutritional supplements you could possibly consume. Eat out three times less a month and buy that killer dress or those golf clubs you've been eyeing. If you travel for work and are forced to eat out, then use the restaurants to your benefit by having them serve you exactly what you want and need. They can even give you items not listed on the menu. Choosing the right restaurant and then making them work a little will pay you many benefits.

Oh, there is one other problem with eating out . . . What control do you have over what exactly goes into the meal being prepared for you? (Hint: we're not talking about any normal food ingredients.) Where have the cook and waiter's hands been right before handling your plate? Who sneezed over it and who should have been home in bed with the flu instead of flipping burgers? **Fact: Many cases of "the flu" and just feeling lousy for several days in actuality are food poisonings obtained while dining in restaurants.** You just weren't sick enough or didn't die from it to be counted as an actual case of food poisoning. Improve your odds in this area of the game of life by retaining more control of your health. Make your own meals and exercise some control over whom you allow to sneeze over your meal!

9. **Remember why you eat.** You don't eat because the dinner bell

rang or because it's just the correct time. If you can realize each time you reach for that Snicker's bar that you eat because of the specific nutritional needs of your body, then you will probably make wiser decisions. A pregnant woman's cravings are probably the best example of the human body's call out for help. The acidity and salt content of the pickle has given this sour treat its reputation with carrying women. Ice cream is popular possibly because it is a good source of protein, calcium and vitamin D.

Don't eat because you're bored, nervous or depressed. Don't eat because it's the lunch hour if you had a big snack at 10:30. Don't eat because you cannot sleep. Stay away from the pantry and the icebox unless your body actually ***needs*** the food. Reach for a glass of filtered water instead. Remember that eating is more than a just a social habit.

Let's add, "**Make it count**" to this category since it is related to the thought of why you eat. If you will make every bite count toward the nutritional needs of your body, then you will again make better choices. A donut gives you nothing in the way of a positive nutritional contribution. An apple, on the other hand, offers several benefits including: fiber, vitamins, minerals and those all-important phytonutrients making it a very powerful snack. There is no comparison between the two. "I'll take two jelly-filled ones, please."

10. **Plant it, Buckwheat!** This is, beyond a doubt, the most important of the guidelines. Move from a meat dominated diet (and society) to one with the emphasis more on plant-based foods. We are not carnivores. Yes, there are many vitamins and minerals found in meats, but a lot less animal meat will still give you what you need and also allow you to live longer. Most meats are hard on your system. They are difficult to digest, contain way too much cholesterol and potentially harmful bacteria, and have really very few benefits to justify such a

significant role in our diet. People that consume absolutely no meat products have shown us that it can be done. Your health will improve by making this change in your diet, even if you make no other changes at all! Most Americans get more protein than they need, so cut back on the meat, make it less of a dinner centerpiece and add quality years to your life.

If you get nothing else from this crucial step to your health and well being, then listen to what Dr. Paul Talalay, the John Jacob Abel Distinguished Service Professor of Pharmacology and Director of the Laboratory for Molecular Sciences at the Johns Hopkins University School of Medicine (Whew! What a long title!) had to say. "The development of cancer is a long, multi-step process that requires many years to complete. For example, it takes as long as thirty years for prostate cancer to develop (even longer in women . . . since they don't even have a prostate gland). We don't know whether the body's defenses will knock out the cancer along the way. **It's far easier to disrupt the process that leads to cancer than to cure the disease after it develops.** I contend that one of the best ways to intervene early is with a proper diet." His research is in a diet rich in fruits and vegetables, and the plant substances called phytochemicals. He's a pretty smart man. Take his advice.

Bonus guideline: pH balance

Even more critical to your body than the narrow span allowed for body temperature differential, the pH level of your blood must remain within a minute range. If not, several things can happen, none of them good. The pH level (potential hydrogen molecules) that most of us are familiar with have to do with pool chemistry. Those of you that have had pools know that if you do not keep the water at close to 7.2 on the pH scale, problems will follow. Too alkaline and the equipment gets gummed up with calcium deposits, too acidic and the equipment can be destroyed and the pool surface literally etched to the point of ruin. Either direction can get very expensive.

Your body's blood supply must remain at approximately 7.4 (slightly alkaline, as 7.0 is neutral), not giving a lot of wiggle-room, even less than your pool chemistry would allow. Your entire metabolic process depends on this slightly alkaline environment. If it becomes too acidic, body tissues corrode, which disrupts and interrupts all cellular functions. Muscle, heart, lung and brain tissues, and all of your organs are adversely affected, ultimately resulting in premature aging and cellular mutations including cancers and all disease.

Your body has a wonderful way of protecting itself. It determines which function is highest in the pecking order of importance and protects that first. (Your blood supply always wins that contest.) Ninety-nine times out of one hundred, the battle that it fights is to maintain alkalinity, since the fuel we give our bodies is usually trying to drag it down to the acid side. This next point may help you understand one aspect of your body's chemistry. All chemicals, minerals and substances on this earth are either acid or alkaline in nature. Calcium is a base (alkaline). When the pH level in your blood drops (becomes acidic) from the acidic foods you eat and you haven't consumed enough calcium with that meal, your system goes right to the pH bank, your bones, and extracts the calcium it needs to bring pH normality to its vital blood supply. Do we perhaps see a problem here? Osteoporosis plus osteoartritis, many nervous system disorders, and all heart disease to name a few of the maladies that come to mind.

Unfortunately, the vast majority of the foods you consumed before beginning this program were acidic. All animal meats, all dairy products, most grains, coffee, alcohol, sugars of any type, unnaturally processed foods, pastas, many fats and Cheese-Wiz are all highly acidic. What foods are alkaline? All vegetables, a few fruits, some nuts and seeds are alkaline. (Water is neutral.) Depressed yet? You need not be. Most of the foods recommended on this program are plant based and thus close to being alkaline. Drinking a lot of water and eating plenty of salads will do much to get your blood pH level where it needs to be.

However, if you are seriously ill and want to get as much out of this program as possible, then, additionally, please read the book, *The pH Miracle,* written by Robert O. Young, Ph.D. and Shelley Redford Young. Dr. and Mrs. Young have spent the last twenty-five years or so researching this topic and they have tied all disease and aging to the level of pH in the blood. The book is chock full of testimonials of people cured from everything from fatigue to cancer by following the very strict regime they outline in their book. It is quite profound reading and if you are not yet on the "garbage in-garbage out" bandwagon, this book may help get you there.

Follow these ten plus guidelines and your health will improve greatly. Again, this is not rocket science, nor is it difficult to understand. It does, however, require some willpower and common sense, but the dividends are huge.

Top Ten Super Foods

By eating certain foods or types of foods, you can insure that you'll be getting the proper mix of nutrients including; vitamins, minerals, fiber and antioxidants along with the correct balance of proteins, fats, and carbohydrates. By concentrating on these, weight loss will be easier to accomplish, trips to the doctor should be minimized and your overall health should improve.

Here is a list of ten foods or food types that should be a part of your weekly diet. There are a variety of reasons for selecting these foods. It may be that they are, as mentioned, good sources of fiber, vitamins, minerals, phytonutrients and/or have other benefits. They will be low in fat, will probably be complex instead of simple carbohydrates, may assist your digestive system and may prevent diseases. These are potent foods, or food groups and it is important for you to make them a part of your life. It may be difficult to fit all of them in on a daily basis, so try and include these as often as is possible.

1. **Yogurt,** preferably nonfat, lite (meaning 25% less calories), and only those containing "active cultures." No, not frozen yogurt! ***This*** yogurt is high in protein, low in carbohydrates (about twenty per serving as compared to fifty for the normal yogurt!) and contains the microorganisms your digestive system desperately needs to function properly. Remember, everything from antibiotics to alcohol have destroyed the friendly little guys roaming around your intestines that assist in the proper digestion and allocation of the fuel necessary for proper bodily function. These little guys will also assist you in being regular; which is important at your age. Yogurt also contains a third of the calcium required daily, vitamins B-12, folic acid and potassium. Yogurt can help keep you in tiptop shape! It is a must. Supercharge your yogurt by adding; acidophilus, lecithin, ground up flaxseed (for omega fatty acids), soymilk and cut-up fruit.
2. **Vegetables and fruits of color** (is that the politically correct way to refer to them?) Generally speaking, most fruits and vegetables that are rich and deep in color contain the highest concentration of the vital nutrients (phytonutrients) that you need to maintain and build your body properly. Some examples are: tomatoes, broccoli, spinach, yams, carrots, apples, bananas, romaine lettuce, onions, etc. **Orange foods** (i.e. cantaloupes and carrots) contain carotenoids such as beta-carotene that reduce oxidizing damage to DNA and stimulate your immune system while fighting cancer-causing conditions in your body. Deep orange color foods can also protect you from the damaging effects of the sun by acting as an internal

sun-block. **Leafy green vegetables** also contain certain types of carotenes along with vitamin C and folic acid. The natural chemical group they contain called isothiocyanates (warning; trying to pronounce this word will cause severe headaches!) help stimulate the production of cancer fighting liver enzymes. In addition, broccoli contains phytochemicals such as flavonoids and phytoestrogens that battle cancer type system breakdowns. **Oranges** and other **orange/yellow** classified citrus fruits are rich in vitamin C, carotenes, folic acid and over sixty different flavonoids that protect cells from damage. The flavonoids in grape juice reduce blood platelet "stickiness" by over 40%, thus reducing dangerous blood clots. Raisins, blue-berries, strawberries, spinach and kale all contain high levels of antioxidants. Tomatoes, watermelon and pink grapefruit, all considered red foods contain lycopene a highly regarded cancer fighting antioxidant. Even ketchup gets the nod here. Garlic, onions, asparagus and chives, considered white/green soldiers, are also rich in flavonoids that protect against cellular damage (which can cause poor reception on your cell phone.) On top of all the benefits of these fruits and vegetables, they are also high in fiber, which lowers cholesterol and the rate of many cancers such as colon cancer. **Include at least five servings minimum of these daily to get the proper mix of body boosters.** Mix it up by adding multiple food colors daily. **The specific vegetable you choose is not as important as the number of different colors you throw onto your plate.** As you can see, you'll need to pay attention to the variety of fresh foods that you consume. Don't eat only carrots three times a day and consider that your daily allotment of veggies. Besides the overall nutrition of these fresh foods, mix up the color to get the best benefits. Also remember not to overcook them or you'll lose many of the antioxidants. In fact, don't cook them at all to get the absolute best bang for your buck. (Again, salads are the easiest avenue to consume raw vegetables.)

3. **Soy.** This is not your father's soy. Like the Buick, soy has evolved. Before you say, "forget it" and skip over this one, listen to the story on soy. Soy fights cholesterol by lowering the level of LDL (bad) cholesterol and your overall cholesterol. You can think of soluble fiber as microscopic scrub brushes cleaning the inside of your arterial walls as it makes it way through your bloodstream. It's a high source of protein without the saturated fats of animal-based foods. Soy products contain protease, a chemical that inhibits estrogen and other hormones that promote cancerous growth plus genistein, another chemical that protects against cancer in many ways. Populations that consume a large amount of soy-based foods have lower cancer rates and higher levels of longevity across the board. I'm not a big fan of tofu, but roasted soybeans are very tasty and vanilla soy milk (my favorite is the Silk brand) is also very good. If you have problems with dairy products, then this soymilk is for you. Soy is absolutely grand for your heart and well worth working some into your diet for that reason, if nothing else.
4. **Nuts** . . . no, not Pee Wee Herman! We're talking about the protein packed little guys that are a healthy alternative to potato chips and other wasteful snacks as long as you practice the principle of moderation. **Although nuts *are* high in fat, at least they are of the monounsaturated kind, which has actually been shown to lower cholesterol.** Remember, fats don't *make* you fat. They also contain minerals such as potassium, magnesium and zinc, vitamin E and a fair amount of fiber. They boost your immune system and reduce your risk of heart disease and cancer. Add a couple of handfuls of nuts daily instead of that candy bar or bag of chips. Just remember moderation and nuts will serve you well.
5. **Beans and legumes.** Does anybody know what the heck a legume is? Well, I looked it up . . . A legume is a plant of the

pea or bean family having a pod that splits when mature; the seeds or pods are then used as a food. There, now we all have learned something new today. Turns out we have been eating legumes and didn't even know it! As we all know, we eat too much meat and other animal products giving us way too much fat and plaque-causing cholesterol. Consuming beans and legumes gives us the protein that we need with little fat and actually helps lower cholesterol because of its fiber content. In fact, legumes contain more protein that any other vegetable. Also, the carbohydrates in beans are released slowly and thus won't spike your blood sugar levels making beans and legumes perfect for fighting diabetes. Since the carbs in this food group are of the complex type, they help to build stamina and endurance. Lecithin, a type of fat that the brain needs to make a chemical messenger or neurotransmitter and folic acid (a B vitamin) are also star players in beans and legumes. Making a pot of beans is also a good excuse to add garlic and onions to your diet. Beans are very filling and can very easily be the main focus of a meal, (and the entertainment following!) bypassing America's unhealthy craving for the saturated fats found in meats. Researchers from Tulane University and the National Heart, Lung, and Blood Institute studied 9600 people over a nineteen-year period and found that those subjects who ate legumes (including peanut butter!) four times weekly were 22% less likely to develop heart disease than those that consumed them once a week or less. **This food is so important to you that Federal guidelines now count legumes as being equivalent to a serving of either produce or meat!** Make a pot of beans, stew some bean soup, eat four-bean salad, snack on some peanuts instead of a candy bar or add beans when you go through the salad bar; any way that you can sneak some "pods" into your diet will reap many rewards. (Use soybeans and double your money!)

6. **Fish.** Omega-3 oils (an essential fatty acid, essential means that your body needs, but cannot produce it, so you must supplement it) found in many different types of cold water fish, inhibit blood clotting and can lower the risk of heart disease, prostate, colon, rectum and ovarian cancers. Fish is high in protein, low in saturated fats and if not fried is a must to be added 2–3 times weekly to your diet. There is a ton of data now praising the omega-3 and omega-6 fatty acids and how consuming both of them can add years to your life. Societies that consume larger amounts of fish than Americans live a heck of a lot longer than we do. (When dining on fish, stay away from the tartar sauce and rich butter preparations to keep this on the healthy side. There are several spices and healthy oils that can be used to add wonderful flavoring.)
7. **Tea.** Green, black and herbal. Take your pick. All three teas have many different benefits to your health and should be a part of your daily regimen. They are full of antioxidants, help regulate blood pressure, cholesterol, and support your immune system. Yes, most of them contain caffeine, but usually much less than a regular cup of coffee. (Most are one half the caffeine of coffee.) Mix it up and substitute teas instead of coffee. Also try herb teas for the specific maladies as they are intended to treat. Green tea has been getting all of the good press recently, but truthfully speaking, black tea, almost 80% percent of all tea produced in the world, has many of the same benefits as the green. In fact, tea leaves of all types may have as many flavonoids as fruits and vegetables. Among its other benefits, black tea has been shown to restore arterial function in patients with arteriosclerosis. Not bad for a simple cup of tea! Green and black teas contain enough fluoride to inhibit tooth decay. One more plus, green tea kills more bacteria in your mouth than mint, parsley *and* chewing gum. If your breath precedes you and leaves a lasting impression, drink green tea!

8. **Garlic and Onions.** Besides keeping vampires and any potential spouses away, these two wonder plants will go into battle for you like no other foods. Garlic, like honey has been used for thousands of years for everything from an aphrodisiac to a cure for hypertension. The ancient Egyptians actually worshipped it for its healing qualities. Louis Pasteur found that garlic was an effective natural antibiotic and was used to treat tuberculosis among other ailments. Allicin, a compound in garlic, helps thin the blood making it a useful treatment for heart disease, clotting disorders and high blood pressure. It also helps lower cholesterol and builds your immune system so that your body can better fight disease on its own. Garlic and onions do approximately the same things. Use garlic and onions as often as you can. Their frequent use has been shown to be extremely useful in many, many studies.
9. **Fresh, pure water.** Without it you cannot survive, pure and simple. Run your auto dry of fluids and you have big problems. Without even knowing you, I'd be willing to bet that you don't get enough water. Instead you drink coffee, soft drinks, caffeine, and alcohol, all of which are diuretics that actually dehydrate your system. **Over 60% of your body is water.** Water is needed in virtually every process or chemical reaction your body goes through. Blood, sweat and tears are water. So are mucus and spit. All cells need water to dissolve toxins and flush them out of your system. Water lubricates your joints, makes your skin supple and cushions your organs. You can use it to help lose weight, build endurance and muscles. **You must continually flush water through your system to stay healthy. This is probably more important than any other health tip that you can use!** Drink at least eight tall glasses of water a day, more if you exercise a lot. Drink one at each of these points of the day and it will be easier to achieve the goal of eight glasses: when you awake, at breakfast, on the way to work, before

lunch, mid day, before dinner and before bed. See, that was easy wasn't it? Distilled water is probably the best way to fulfill your requirement. However, that's not usually practical, so drink filtered water if you can. If not, just drink. "Okay, where'd I put my beer?"

10. **Whole grains.** These have already been discussed previously, but since we have such a preoccupation with breads, you're going to eat them regardless. Just make your choices primarily whole grain, and at least you'll be satisfying an actual bodily need while consuming them. These not only allow you to get fiber and several vitamins along the way, they taste a heck of a lot better, too. Our society, as a whole, eats way too much bread and you should attempt to reduce the amount that you consume on a daily basis. It's not difficult to cut your allotment to one or two servings a day.

There are plenty of other foods that can be of huge benefit to you that can help jumpstart you on your way to increased longevity, including most of the fruits and vegetables on this planet. These include: lean chicken, low fat dairy products, certain pastas, long grain rice, red wine, and other alcohol in moderation only (darn), soups and some cereals. Use the common sense that you now possess and make wise decisions.

Ten No-No Foods

Julia Child once said, "For every food, there is an equal and opposite food." That timely quote came from . . . I can't seem to find the source right now, I'll have to get back to you on that one.

There are certainly sociological and psychological reasons for eating (we have a multibillion dollar restaurant industry to prove that), **but the main reason that you are *supposed* to consume food is to supply your body with the nutrients and fluids that it needs**

to function properly. It needs proteins, carbohydrates and fats. As previously mentioned, the vita in the word vitamin means essential in Latin, and vitamins *are* just that. You also require dozens and dozens of minerals like potassium and calcium that are needed in abundance, to zinc and selenium that only require trace amounts. The key word is "required." These are all absolutely necessary for proper functioning and are crucial to live a long and energetic life.

What happens when you consume nutritionally deficient foods (those with little or no nutritional value otherwise known as "junk food")? Your body doesn't get what it needs, so it wants more. Couldn't this be a major reason we overeat? Even though there is no conscious thought process telling you that you might as well have put cardboard down your throat, there are many signals sent causing you to eat, eat and eat more. Eventually your body just assumes that you're not getting the message and it decides to punish you by adding layers of fat where you least want the extra baggage. If you're really bad, it will take away your sex drive...all of it! Then all you are left with is your appetite and a propensity to watch daytime TV.

So although much of the empty-calorie foods taste good, your primary job is to give yourself what you need, not just what you want. The following is a list of the ten food types to avoid on a regular basis because they are doing nothing for you except adding bulk to your diet and waistline. You do not have to exclude these permanently (that would be asking too much!); just avoid them whenever possible. However, if you're excessively heavy, then you will need to stay away from them as though they were telemarketers until you get a head start on taking off the excess poundage.

Remember that these foods do you absolutely no good as far as supplying the nutrition your body needs to run properly and efficiently and in fact probably will do you plenty of harm by either spiking your blood sugar level too fast or will be stored around your waist for future use as a cushion.

1. **White sugar.** As empty as Leon Spinks' head with blood sugar level spikes that look similar to the NASDAQ! Think of cotton candy and colas. These should be labeled as poison . . .
2. **White flour.** We Americans have this obsession with white and pure as though they are clean and good. Clean, yes. In fact, white flour is so clean that it has been bleached, cooked and stripped of all its nutritional value. (Same goes with white sugar.) You're left with only the simple carbohydrates that enters your system too fast, spiking your insulin and blood sugar levels eventually causing such minor problems as: diabetes, heart disease, obesity and high blood pressure! All the nutrients are washed away, and it hasn't given your body anything of value except for maybe taste. And since it enters your blood system quicker, it actually make you hungry again sooner than if you consumed slower digesting whole grain complex carbohydrates found in whole grain wheat breads.
3. **Fried foods.** Not much explanation is necessary. Abounding in saturated fats and trans fatty acids. Consider them "the plague"!
4. **Soft drinks.** Triple whammy! The sugar in soft drinks is of the insulin-spiking type, the caffeine revs up your metabolism while actually dehydrating your cells, and on top of that most soft drinks contain a preservative called phosphoric acid that will leach the calcium out of your bones. (Phosphorus needs to remain balanced with calcium in your bloodstream. Get too much phosphorus and your system pulls the calcium it needs to restore that balance out of storage . . . your bones.) One Harvard study showed that teenage girls who drank sodas regularly were more apt to break bones than those who didn't. Many of them are already showing the beginning signs of osteoporosis, and they weren't even out of puberty yet. Cut way down on your consumption of soft drinks in general. Drink nonfat milk, water, tea or juices and if you must, limit your usage tremendously. For every cola that you drink, you are

eliminating one glass of water that you will be unable to drink for feeling full.

5. **Animal fats.** An occasional steak or burger won't kill you, but this obsession with meat at every evening meal is not healthy. First of all, if you're going to consume meat at all, it should be for breakfast or lunch, when you actually need it. The proteins will be used more during the day than at night. On top of being high in cholesterol and saturated fats they are hard to digest making nighttime sleep more labored. Put them on a grill and you get the added bonus of ingesting a few carcinogens. Center meals around salads instead of meats, and that alone will improve your health tremendously.
6. **Excessive alcohol.** A drink or two probably won't hurt and may actually be of benefit to the majority of us. More than that on a fairly regular basis can and will do damage. **Besides dehydrating your system, an overuse of alcohol will trash your liver and, if prolonged, will lead to diabetes, heart disease, liver or related cancers and premature death.** Without sounding like a "tea totaller," it is safe to say that **alcohol abuse is one of the top preventable health problems in the United States.** Not only does it lead to physical health problems to the person doing the drinking, it usually hurts the people around them. Spousal and child abuse because of alcohol are a lot more prevalent (and usually hidden) than we as a society want to talk about. The collateral damage to our nation is out of control. There is work-related down time and productivity issues, hospitalization costs, drunk driving accidents and families being torn apart because of alcohol. It is everywhere and can only be controlled by you taking back your health and sanity. You that have an alcohol problem know who you are. Get it under control for the good of everyone in and around your life. Alcohol and cigarettes are similar. They both kill you and injure the people around you, just using different styles.

7. **Excessive caffeine.** Caffeine is everywhere. It's in most colas whether diet or not, coffee and coffee drinks, teas and chocolates. Pretty much your entire diet! A serving or two is beneficial, more than that can give you blood pressure problems, constrict your blood vessels, and diminish the effects of your immune system allowing cancers to get a foothold inside of you. Too much caffeine increases urinary excretion taking excess calcium out of your system. It's rough on pregnant women, can cause some unneeded anxiety and will dehydrate you. Moderate use shows many benefits including: increased energy and awareness levels, protection against certain diseases including Parkinson's and some cancers and of course positive social implications. However, to get the benefits, limit your overall daily intake to no more than 2–3 servings daily and avoid caffeine later than mid-afternoon so as to not disturb your sleeping habits. Again, moderation is the key.
8. **Candies.** An occasional candy may help curb your craving, but can rot your teeth and eventually add excessive calories to your diet. You're better off with sugarless gum (avoid those sweetened with aspartame) that will help your digestive system get going and that can actually increase your metabolic rate by the chewing action. One small candy several times daily will sneak your calorie count upwards more than you realize.
9. **Creamed foods.** Again, if it tastes too good to be true, it is probably not good for you. Usually anything creamy has gotten that way by using ingredients counterproductive to a healthy diet. Cream dressings, gravy, pasta sauces and salads can be brutal. Try substituting Italian dressing, pesto sauce, nonfat yogurt for mayonnaise and avoid potato salad and coleslaw. You'll save plenty of calories. If it's creamy, it ain't dreamy.
10. **Too much of any one type of food.** Variety is the key to any good diet. If you use up all your daily calorie intake on a couple of foods types then you're probably not getting all the vitamins,

mineral and antioxidants that your body needs. Mix it up. Eat vegetables and fruits. Eat proteins, fats and carbohydrates. Don't fill up on breads and other starches. Salads are excellent for your health but don't eat one at every meal. You'll get tired of it and may not get the variety that you need. Again, moderation plays a key role. Consume 2,000 calories of pizza and there is not much room left for anything else.

TOTALLY ORGANIC, DUDE

Should you eat only organic foods? It depends. If it will make you feel better, if it is relatively easy to find and not too expensive, if it is easy to prepare and of course, if it tastes good, go ahead. Theoretically speaking, organic foods should be better for you. For instance, organically grown fruits and vegetables should be totally free of pesticides, right? Well, they're not. USDA tests have shown that while conventionally grown produce contains pesticide residue 73% of the time, organically grown fruits and vegetables did so in 23% of the tested samples. Why? Either mislabeling of the produce or pesticide runoff and/or over-spraying from conventional fields probably accounted for the bulk of their findings. Organics are much better for you, but are far from ideal.

As far as processed foods using organically grown foods, the choice is yours. Let your taste buds and pocket books decide.

It is fairly easy to get rid of most of the residue from conventionally grown produce, and organically grown foods as well. Just wash them with diluted dish soap or baking soda and rinse completely, then peel or prepare as you would normally. If you scrub apples, potatoes and other hard surface produce and soak strawberries, blueberries and other softer foods, that should be sufficient to eliminate the vast majority of the toxins that you ingest. Hopefully your stomach, immune system and liver will take care of the rest. This may seem contradictory to the idea of getting rid of all toxins that you encounter, but making this program more difficult and harder to follow is counter productive. You very much need to stay on this path and making your food choices tough to adhere to doesn't help any. Overall, organics are probably better for you. There are antibiotic and hormone issues with conventional animal meats. Organically grown produce should have a higher mineral content from using the soil better, so use your own judgment. There is labeling requirements just signed into law that may help raise the overall quality of organic foods available. If organics are readily available and cost effective, then choose them.

Bad Data

There are a couple of observations that can be made concerning studies and research done on food and supplements. Since you now know that there are vast differences in the efficiency of the typical American's digestive system, it can be assumed that the fuel brought in may or may not be assimilated with the same efficiency. In other words, different people have a varying degree of absorption of all nutrients taken into their bodies. **Because of this, most studies done to judge the benefit of certain foods, vitamins, minerals and other supplements consumed by the American public are flawed at best. How can one say whether a substance does or does not work when the mechanics of the body used in the study does not consistently react the same?** As an example, if all of a study's subjects take in and absorb selenium differently, how is the effectiveness of the selenium judged? Not very accurately, I would say.

Take any one single study lightly before you jump to conclusions. If there are several studies all pointing to selenium being of benefit to your health in some way, then go ahead and add it to your daily regime. The same goes for foods. The tomato, for instance, has tons of data showing that consuming them on a regular basis will be of benefit to your health, so go ahead and assume that this delicious food will help you. This is especially true once you improve the efficiency of your digestive system by taking the steps outlined in this program. If a certain food offers some benefit to a limited number of people, then you will probably be included in that short list, because your system will absorb nutrients more efficiently. You'll basically get more bang for your buck out of the food and supplements that you consume.

It's obvious that people care for themselves differently and will not get the same benefit from the foods that they eat. So it's in your best interest to have a healthy diet that will help fuel your body's needs and maximize your health potential.

Located in our newspaper is a comic strip titled *Hermann*. You have probably seen it from time to time. One was particularly funny. Hermann is talking to his wife at a restaurant, lamenting to her the importance of eating properly. He said, "You know, you are what you eat." Just then, the waitress comes to take their order and Hermann replies, "I'll have the boneless, skinless chicken breast." Of course, his wife just stared at him and smiled.

You really are what you eat. At least the end result is dependant upon what you put into your mouth. In order to maximize your efficiency, you'll need to monitor very carefully what you eat. It doesn't have to be boring, though. There are many wonderful foods and dishes that will do the trick. Make the right decisions and the results will speak for themselves. Just don't expect any miracles in too short of time. Stay away from junk and move toward a plant-based diet. Cut down on your portion sizes and eat different colored foods on a regular basis. Drink plenty of water, tea and avoid sweetened beverages. Re-establish the bacteria that need to be thriving in your intestinal tract. Wash the pesticides from your fresh fruits and vegetables and eat them as close to raw as possible. If you must have starchy foods, stick to whole grains and keep them to a minimum. You won't have any trouble reaching your daily requirement of carbohydrates! Eat fresh fish, soy products, beans and occasionally lean meat. Don't eat processed or creamy foods. Limit your sit-down and fast-food restaurant experiences and when you do go, "have it your way" or go elsewhere. Remember, the only one regulating what goes down your hatch is you. *Bon Appetite!*

Step 5:

Insurance

Not too terribly long ago, the World Trade Center towers in New York City were permanently erased from our American landscape causing one of those "life changing," and in this case "society changing" experiences, forever altering America as Pearl Harbor did some 60 years ago. Stressing the importance of getting enough fiber in our diets sometimes doesn't seem all that important . . .

America is the greatest country in the entire history of the world. That's not boastful, only truthful. We are the most modern and technologically advanced. We invent, patent, copyright, build, grow and manufacture a majority of the world's needs. Medicines developed here are used to save the lives of millions of people around the entire globe. The vast majority of the creative and forward-thinking minds call America their home. Our economy is so dominating that any ripple in its seam is felt around the world.

What makes us so great? What makes us perform as well as we have done for so many years, so many decades? Our freedom and the opportunities provided because of that freedom are the first things that come to mind. Not too far behind that has to be our overall health, because without that we would have nothing. We wouldn't think as well, we wouldn't have the energy and the enthusiasm needed to carry out our destinies, and we wouldn't have the tolerance or the patience required to allow the expression of the many freedoms provided for in our wonderful, but imperfect constitution. We wouldn't have the energy or the capacity to love ourselves, the ones around us, or have compassion for total strangers on the other side of the world. Our lifestyle, diet and environment all contribute to that well-being. However, over the past fifty years or so, we have taken our wonderful diet for granted, decimating the nutritional value of the foods we consume in the name of convenience and speed. As a result, our diet has changed drastically and we are no longer supplying our bodies with what they need to function properly. Before this trend leads to the total breakdown of our systems and ultimately our competitive edge in the world, we-as a nation-need to get a handle on our health.

In order to return to a level of good health, you need to take precautions; you need an insurance policy for your precious body. Improving your diet is not enough by itself. You need some help, and supplements are just that. Taking the proper nutrients will assure that you are giving your body what it requires to carry out the great things that you are capable of accomplishing.

Since we don't live in a perfect dietary world, supplements, in general, are necessary to maintain an optimal level of efficiency in the human body. As was mentioned in the chapter about diet, our ancestors got what they needed from the vitamin and mineral-rich fresh foods they ate, the pure water they drank and they were not bombarded with all of the harmful environmental forces we are subjected to today. Many of our present day issues include: dirty air, polluted waters, chemically treated and otherwise processed foods and the multitude of stresses on our systems caused by the pressures of today's society. All of these put an enormous strain on your entire body. This, by itself, should be an obvious reason to make sure that you are running a finely tuned machine.

Our predecessors had plenty of health dilemmas of their own such as an overall ignorance about smoking and pesticide uses, saturated fat consumption, lack of vaccinations and the unavailability of today's wonderful medical breakthroughs. Our grandparents, if they made it past childbirth (which was a gamble by itself!), had a much shorter life span than we will have today, and they probably died fairly sudden by today's standards. They suffered from a major lack of the technology available now that would have kept them going or cured what ailment they had. They simply didn't know what we do today. **Although we are certainly living longer today, that doesn't necessarily mean that the quality of that additional living is that much better than before.** Keeping someone alive for ten extra years doesn't say much if the quality of life isn't very good. What good does it do to live those extra years if you're crippled with arthritis, can't breath easily because of pulmonary emphysema, a trip to the store wears you out or cancer is eating away at your very life? We can very easily live longer than our parents. One of the goals of this program is to ensure that not only do you live longer, but that your quality of life is also better than that of your ancestors.

Can you imagine what you could have done for some of your deceased relatives with some simple vaccines available at your local pharmacy today? What if you had been able to get your grandfather on a walking program and convinced him to quit smoking? **The possibilities are endless, but what you cannot do for your dead relatives you can do for yourself.** By taking advantage of what we have learned so far and using some of the good common-sense precautions that may have been buried or forgotten long ago, you can have an exceptional lifestyle till the end. A bonus being that maybe, just maybe, you can pass some of that wisdom on to your children . . . Well, *that* might be asking for too much!

We are going to lump many different types of substances together into a bundle called **supplements.** We'll combine: herbs, minerals, vitamins, chemicals, enzymes and even foods that aren't usually considered foods into this basket. That may not be scientifically correct, but will serve our purpose of simplicity. However, they do have one important characteristic in common that is crucial to understand and that concerns the method that most of them work under. Take a couple of aspirin and your headache will go away shortly. Swallow a muscle relaxer and your back spasm may stop fairly quickly. Begin taking the herb saw palmetto and you may *never* notice any change. It may very well keep you (men) from contracting prostate cancer, but you probably won't notice anything the entire time you take the herb. Take vitamin C and you may not notice any change happening to your body. That's okay, though, because vitamin C may keep you from getting a cold or a flu bug, and that's when you would change from being fine to feeling rotten.

What most supplements are designed to do is to put your body in a position to heal itself. Supplements feed and build your immune system, allow your blood to flow better or keep your blood pressure and cholesterol levels under control. They contain antioxidants that search out and destroy harmful cellular malfunctions, substances that nuke cancerous bodies in your blood, or they work with your body to remove the underlying cause of a variety of illnesses. The noticeable change, if any, may be subtle.

That, unfortunately, is not acceptable in today's world of instant gratification. You take a pill today and you want to see results before going to bed. Try and remember that your body was designed to take care of itself. All you have to do is feed and take care of it properly and it will do the rest. Give your insides what it needs and, by design, it will perform magnificently. Plus, it has taken twenty to thirty years for you to screw things up. It will take some time to straighten out your entire system and change the momentum of your health from poor to good. Supplements are an excellent means of accomplishing that goal.

There is literally no disease called "old age." Other than some terrible accident, you will die from: a physical breakdown in your immune system, a weakness or failure in another system within your body or the constant nagging of your children, whichever comes first. You won't die from "old age." Supplements, whether directly or indirectly will target your immune system in general, and help your body fight the many forces bombarding it hundreds of times daily every day of your life.

Most of the substances that you can supplement your diet with today are not new. In fact, many of them have been around and shown to be effective for thousands of years. Ginseng, ginkgo, garlic, ginger, honey and vinegar have been around forever. The Chinese have been using herbs and other supplements to treat virtually every ailment known to them for over five thousand years. That should be a long enough period of time to decide whether or not something is of value to the human body. If ginkgo biloba wasn't useful, they would have dropped it from their bag of goodies long ago. But the Chinese philosophy is different from ours. They revere the human body, understand the balance that is needed in life and take steps to insure that their bodies are strong enough to endure the challenges that it faces. They don't get a shot every time they feel sick. Instead, they try to restore the balance in a particular system by feeding it herbs, plants or other foods it needs. Their culture has been around a lot longer than ours and will probably outlast ours. There are many truths to be said about respecting the wisdom of your elders and as societies go, the Chinese are our elders.

Some substances are fairly new, or at least recently discovered and don't have the track record that many herbs have. For those, like glucosamine sulfate, you'll have to rely on the studies done and your common sense to decide whether or not it is right for you. There are many sources to research the effectiveness of supplements, whether through the internet, periodicals, published studies, health food and other book stores, your doctor and even your newspaper. Find a health practitioner, whether it is your doctor or some other forward-thinking health expert and get their input. Read, ask questions and use your common sense to make some very important decisions about your life. Don't just shovel pills down your throat. Do the research and make the right choices.

The Players

Understanding the roles of the following players is crucial for you to fully appreciate the importance of supplements. There are two different types of players when discussing the role that supplements play in your overall health. Basically, it's the good versus the bad, the offense versus the defense, the democrats versus the republicans, the cowboys versus the Indians and the attorneys versus the . . . the . . . versus everyone else. Most supplements are designed to give your body the tools to fight all the negative influences that it gets bombarded with (that would be the bad guys), whether it's from inside your body or outside of your skin. The supplements that you take will either use the nutrients they have to directly attack the harmful elements or they will assist your body in producing some other protector (acting as enzymes) to fight those all important battles.

First, we'll introduce the visiting team, the cannibals, Ivan the Terrible, Irving the Horrific, the cowboys in black hats better known as **"The Bad Guys."** Very creative names, wouldn't you say?

"The Bad Guys"

Free Radicals.

(Not Abbie Hoffman.) Free radicals are actually oxygen atoms that cause damage to your cells. Most normal atoms have stable pairs of electrons. Free radical atoms have one electron missing and nature doesn't like that. One of the reasons it is missing the electron is the result of the energy metabolism of your cells. It is similar to your car's exhaust, a natural bi-product of combustion. So, what does it do? It goes out and steals one from a nearby atom, which in turn causes *that* atom to now be unstable. A domino effect then occurs causing more free radical electrons to search out and damage other healthy cells. It is a vicious cycle. **This occurs all the time. If this happens *too* often, and is not kept in check by your immune system, the resulting damage can be catastrophic to your body. Your cell's DNA can become mutated and a myriad of different things can happen, none of them good. The result of these reactions will eventually compromise your immune system leading to infection, various degenerative diseases and will certainly speed up your overall aging process, even if it doesn't cause any life-threatening illnesses.**

Cancer also gets its start in the bowels of this hideous player, while two good examples of degenerative diseases are arthritis and heart disorders. There are several types of free radicals (some of them are actually beneficial), but one of the main culprits hangs around the oxygen molecule. You already know that oxidation can ruin your automobile. It causes rust and can "total" your car. The same holds true inside of you, except you don't exactly rust!

The oxygen form of the free radical causes a lot of the damage to the human body. It's ironic that we need oxygen to live, but present oxygen in the wrong environment and it can literally kill you. **Since oxidation occurs more readily in fat molecules, a diet high in the wrong kinds of fat can and will lead to permanent**

damage to your system. (This demonstrates one more reason to cut down on your fat consumption, especially animal fats.) Eliminate Mr. Free Radical and you eliminate most diseases and ailments. By the way, he has made his respective all-star team every year for the past fifty years. He is at the top of his game and your goal is to strike him out or stop him from reaching first base. Containment is the key. By eating right, taking supplements and keeping your immune system in tip-top shape, you have the best chance of taking Mr. Radical out of the game.

Other than losing big at the casino, most of the problems that you will face as you age have to do with free radical damage to your cells. All of the wrong behaviors, like a poor diet, hanging around environmental poisons such as petroleum bi-products and politicians, not exercising and smoking all contribute to free-radical production. Your assignment, if you choose to accept it, is to keep down the total number of free radicals in your system. You cannot eliminate them completely since some are good and every time you stick something in your mouth you create free radicals. Just maintaining the proper balance will do.

"Supporting Cast"

The other bad players are: pollutants, pesticides, tobacco smoke, ultraviolet light, radiation, grunge music and other poisons of all types and don't really need to be discussed here. (You know who they are. In fact, you can see their "mugs" at your local Post Office and you should already recognize their insidious behavior.) The appetite of the bad players motivates them to team up with Mr. Free Radical to cause cancers and nervous system disorders like Parkinson's and Alzheimer's. With a little conscience effort, you can stay away from and eliminate them from making a contribution toward your funeral . . . (Well, maybe you can let them bring a covered dish or something else as long as they promise not to infect any of your mourners.)

"THE GOOD GUYS"

Now, introducing . . . **The Good Guys!!!** This team is your first and final defense against the negative influences your system sees thousands of times each and every day. You would not be alive today without these team players. In fact, you wouldn't even have made it out of infancy. Unfortunately, as you age, the job (the number of harmful players) becomes harder to manage and the good guys' presence in your body is diminished by several factors. Most of them centering around the abuses you have previously put your body through. The Good Guys' lineup is as follows:

Antioxidants

Antioxidants chase down the free radicals (oxygen type) and tie them up (literally) rendering them useless until they can be flushed out of your system. A more formal definition is that they are nutrients that possess the capacity to chemically react with and neutralize harmful molecules. In effect, they neutralize the damaging free radicals. There are now several hundred different types of antioxidants that have been identified. They can be specific vitamins, minerals or enzymes and travel throughout your body hunting down free radicals. You have heard them being mentioned with several of the foods that contain them. Beta carotene is a good example of an antioxidant and is also a carotenoid (described next.) If a certain food contains antioxidants, you can bet that it has at least some benefit to you.

Carotenoids

Carotenoids are related to the manufacturing of vitamin A. Some are antioxidants and some are part of the actual building process of vitamin A. All of them, which are found in fruit and vegetables, help to fight disease. When you think of carrots, think of rich color and carotenoids.

Phytochemicals

Over 4,000 of these have been found in vegetables, fruits, legumes (beans) and even coffee and tea. These substances are responsible for giving plants their color, flavor and natural disease resistance. That last trait is what concerns humans. They can play a major role in your fight against diseases through improving your immune system. They will fight cancer by blocking one or more of the steps that a cell takes before it becomes cancerous.

Phytochemicals come in many different forms and perform slightly different functions depending up the food that they are found in, but all of them help to prevent diseases of one kind or another. Hundreds of different studies have all shown the positive effects of phytochemicals in the human body. Remember to eat a variety of fresh colorful foods and you'll get all that you need!

Flavonoids

Flavonoids are a popular type of phyto-chemical found in fruits and berries among other places. They also give their hosts its bright colors. This antioxidant cancer-beater prevents cancerous particles from latching onto your cells before they can get a foothold. There are over 400 different types of flavonoids, all of them doing essentially the same thing. They will fight to the death defending your body against cancer.

Amino Acids

Protein, the second most abundant substance in your body (water being first), is essential to all phases of the proper functioning of your system. It's another one of those "without it, you die" ingredients. Protein is essential to life, period. The molecular building blocks of protein are amino acids. **Besides building protein molecules, amino acids play important roles in the production of hormones, enzymes and other aspects of your**

immune system. You liver makes about 80% of the necessary amino acids. The remainder must come from your diet. Some of the proteins you may of heard of are lysine, tryptophan, and phenylalanine. You can find many ways to supplement these through foods, protein drinks, vitamins, etc.

Vitamins

Vitamins, obviously on the Good Guy team, are organic compounds that your body requires for almost all of your life-sustaining functions. They are needed for metabolism, growth, creating hormones and enzymes and for the most part **cannot be manufactured by your body alone.** There are thirteen vitamins and all of them are essential to your body.

Some are water-soluble, which means that they can't be stored in your system for very long. They end up being flushed out of your body as a normal part of your cleansing process. Vitamin C and all of the B-vitamins are examples of these. The others are the fat-soluble type which are stored in your liver and fatty tissue for later use. **Vitamins A, D, E and K are of fat-soluble vitamins, which also need to be taken with a fat for proper absorption, a very important point to remember when swallowing these.**

Note: The following explanations for all of the supplements are going to be fairly brief for the obvious chapter and time restrictions. Because of that, 90% of all the benefits listed are either based in hard facts, countless studies, recent discoveries or common sense. There will be no wild claims, no guarantees, no magic pills or potions. In general, all of these are important to your well being and should not be ignored.

Vitamin A — named for the . . . named for the first letter of the alphabet. (Hey, it could have been worse. It could have been called vitamin #1.) Vitamin A is the "eye" vitamin because it can, among other things, help to prevent night blindness. It actually helps your epithelial tissues (what?) which are the cells that make up your skin, line your eyes, nose, mouth, throat, lungs, etc. It also helps your immune system, can prevent ulcers, protects against cancer and other pollutants, aids in the formation of bones and teeth, and protects you against colds and the flu. Vitamin A is an antioxidant and is related to (on its father's side) carotenoids, the most popular (as voted by the other vitamins) being beta-carotene. The carotenoids should be a crucial aspect of your diet for building a strong immune system. If you eat a good balanced diet you shouldn't have a vitamin A deficiency. However, if you want to make sure you're getting enough vitamin A, the following foods are good sources; animal livers (yuk!), green and yellow fruits and vegetables, and many herbs. Do you remember discussing the colorful foods? Spinach, sweet potatoes, garlic, apricots, asparagus (another yuk), pumpkin, and of course carrots all contain the "eye" vitamin.

B vitamins — There are eight B vitamins and four other related substances that can be grouped in with the Bs. **The water-soluble Bs are the "nerve" vitamins, but perform many other specific and general functions.** They help your cells grow and reproduce properly. They help maintain your nerves, eyes, hair, skin, liver, brain functions, and maintain healthy muscle tone in your intestines. They also help produce the energy that you need to exist by assisting in the breaking down of the foods you consume into a useable substance. The Bs must be consumed together to work properly (it's a union thing). In other words, taking massive B-12 shots won't do you much good if you are deficient in any of the other B vitamins. They don't have to be taken at exactly the same time or amounts, but must all be consumed on a regular daily basis to keep you healthy. The Bs are as follows:

Vitamin B-1, called Thiamine. Ms. Thiamine was born and raised right here in Trenton, New Jersey and hopes to study geology in school after saving the world. Ms. Thiamin assists your circulation and related blood formation, helps produce one of your stomach acids, facilitates carbohydrate metabolism and is one of the primary nerve soldiers. She's also an antioxidant, keeping at bay the effects of aging. (Now don't go out and buy a truck full of Thiamin thinking that it's the proverbial fountain of youth. **You can overdose on most of the B vitamins including thiamine. More is not necessarily better in the vitamin category**). Sources of Vitamin B-1 are: whole grains, wheat germ, fish, egg yolks, meat products, poultry, raisins, sunflower seeds, oatmeal and brown rice. Thiamine can also be found in these herbs; alfalfa, brewers yeast, cayenne, chamomile, peppermint and sage. There are way too many sources of Thiamine to list all of them. Again, eat a balanced diet and you won't have any problems.

Vitamin B-2 — Riboflavin was named after the great thespian, Fred Riboflavin. Mr. Riboflavin is absolutely necessary for red blood cell formation, cellular growth and can help prevent and treat cataracts in your eyes. One of its main functions is in assisting your body in energy production at the cellular level. In fact, without this vitamin you would probably cease to live. But why sweat those minor details!

You need to watch your levels of riboflavin if you exercise a lot, if you take antidepressants or if you suffer from diabetes. You need more of it when you get older *and* if you don't digest milk products well. It may also help with the treatment of carpal tunnel syndrome, eliminate dandruff and help you pick winning lottery numbers. You can find Mr. Riboflavin in: meats, milk products such as cheese and yogurt, egg yolk, poultry, spinach, whole grains, avocados, broccoli, nuts, enriched flour and a variety of other vegetables. Herbs with riboflavin include; alfalfa, cayenne, ginseng, chamomile, sage and red clover. This very important vitamin works hand in hand with some of the other Bs to keep you going strong. A real team player.

Vitamin B-3 — Niacin, also known as the Greek god of wind surfing (discovered deep in King Tut's pyramid in 1904), is the consummate team player. He has led the Knicks in assists for the last eight years and has been their most consistent player since Ewing left! Niacin is similar in characteristics to many of the other Bs. It is needed for good circulation, healthy skin, and makes an enzyme that helps break down carbohydrates into energy. In all it assists in over 50 different processes within your cute little body, but one of the best uses it may have is that it can help lower cholesterol, a huge problem in today's donut-filled world. Find niacin in many of the same foods mentioned in the previous Bs, but to get any cholesterol assistance you will need to get many times the RDA, which is about 12-20 milligrams. Excessive amounts of niacin probably won't hurt you, but may cause your face to flush. Be careful anyway. Find it naturally in brewer's yeast, broccoli, peanuts, tomatoes, wheat germ, alfalfa, parsley, fish, milk products and many other healthy foods.

Vitamin B-5 — Pantothenic Acid is a close cousin to the acid called LSD . . . just kidding! This is the anti-stress vitamin. It works hand in hand with the production of the adrenal hormones, aids in vitamin utilization, converts the foods you eat into energy and is involved in the production of neurotransmitters. It can also enhance your stamina. Yes, that includes sex, too! As you can see, all of the B vitamins are inter-related and B-5 is no exception. You can find pantothenic acid in many foods including whole wheat, beef, vegetables, eggs and brewers yeast.

Vitamin B-6 — This element is know as pyridoxine, or pyro if you happen to be on first name basis with him. Pyridoxine gets around pretty well. He is involved in more bodily functions than Dennis Rodman, and just about any other single nutrient consumed. It helps regulate your sodium/potassium balance, which in turn controls water retention. It is involved in the formation of red blood cells, aids in the functioning of your immune system, acts as a mild diuretic **and** relieves the symptoms of PMS (which may qualify it for the Nobel Peace Prize by itself.)

Allergies, asthma, and arthritis are also relieved by B-6. Again, many of the same sources of the other B-vitamins are the same sources that you can find this crucial element.

Vitamin B-9 — The stage name of this vitamin is folic acid. He never goes by his given name because he is most likely still reeling from the bad PR he received when it was discovered that the American diet was badly lacking of this essential element. The government then required food manufacturers to add folic acid back into the breads, cereals and other products that the manufacturers originally stripped out of many decades earlier. Makes a lot of sense, doesn't it? Folic acid is extremely important in the production of new red blood cells, which take the place of the old and worn out ones headed for the junkyard. In fact, the other cells that wear out quickly, like skin cells and the lining of your intestines also need folic acid. This guy stops birth defects, heart disease and many cancers, but don't worry. You're probably getting enough.

Vitamin B-12 — Cyanocobalamin, or cobalamin. Okay, just call him B-12. You are probably familiar with B-12 shots, sublingual (under the tongue) supplements and other over-the-counter items. They are taken for a burst of energy, though short lived, and for metabolic control (dieting aids). It has many other uses, though. B-12 assists in making healthy red blood cells, it protects your nerve cells, is required for proper digestion, maintains fertility and may help you remember your anniversary. The sources of this vitamin are slightly different than the other Bs in that it's mainly available in meat products. So, if you are a strict vegetarian, you may need B-12 supplements. However, it's also available in dairy products, brewers yeast, kelp, and soybean products. If you are on a restricted diet, you'll need to make a special effort to supplement B-12.

B-Vitamin relatives — Choline, inositol, biotin and PABA are close in nature to the B-vitamins, but have no required daily allowances. (They were also left out of the will of Father "B" when he died and have since filed suit in federal court in an attempt to get some respect from their B cousins.) Since you can't really be deficient in these because they are in most of the foods you consume, we'll just review them briefly. Choline is required for proper nerve transmission and is beneficial in the treatment of Parkinson's disease and other nervous system disorders. Inositol and choline work together to actually make neurotransmitters and move fats out of your liver. Your healthy intestinal bacteria makes biotin, which is needed to properly use the amino acids and fats that you ingest. PABA is a 15-year-old pop singer from Ohio with the current hit song entitled, *Don't rain on my parade, bitch!* In her spare time, PABA, a relative of folic acid, protects you against the earth's elements including sunburns, skin cancer and overcrowded malls. You can find Ms. PABA in whole grains.

Well, that's it for the B-vitamins. **You probably won't need any specific B supplements if you do two things: One, take a good multi-vitamin and two, eat well by including whole grains, soy products, fresh fruits and raw or lightly cooked vegetables in your diet. Consume meat and dairy products wisely. (Wisely translates to "not very much at all.") You may also want to take alfalfa tablets (just about the best all-round supplement there is). You can also use nutritional brewer's yeast as a topping on popcorn or in salads. It gives food a nutty flavor and actually tastes good. Both of those are great B supplements and can be found in most health stores.** Note: if you have pets, add brewer's yeast to their food and you'll never have a problem with their coats, fleas or overall health again.

Vitamin C — Otherwise known as ascorbic acid. This is the Babe Ruth of vitamins, the Tiger Woods of helpful elements. It's also the "mother-in-law" of health, being that you take it for granted most of the time. You don't need much to live on. It doesn't take a lot to keep you from getting scurvy, which is more prevalent in poor countries than in ours. However, if you know how important vitamin C is, then maybe you'll make sure that you are getting more than enough of it to keep you healthy. C is one of your body's top antioxidants, meaning that it searches out and destroys free radicals. These free radicals are the ones roaming around your system looking to wreck havoc on your internal organs, much like your kids. C keeps you from getting cancer, it is necessary to grow and repair tissue, is needed to manufacture collagen (the glue that holds your skeleton and bones together), and can help lessen the common cold. It's the star of your immune system, aids its friends over in the vitamin B section, protects against infection, and can even help lower your blood pressure. (It has also starred in a porn movie several years ago and was also responsible for the last bull-run in the stock market.) C is very diverse, to say the least.

There is a problem with C though; it is water-soluble. So, if you take your mega-dose of C early in the morning, by noon it may have already found a way out of your system. A supplement of 1,000-milligrams a day is better taken as two 500-mg. tablets twice instead of one 1,000-mg mega-pill. Ester-C seems to be the best answer to this particular problem. This type of supplement (actually called esterified for the process . . . wonder if my Aunt Esther had anything to do with it?) is combined with calcium and other minerals that you also need. This special treatment of vitamin C will stay in your system much longer than if you took a ordinary tablet and is many times more potent than normal. If you smoke, have diabetes, allergies or asthma, are sick with the cold or flu, just had surgery, or your spouse's deadbeat brother and his "whacked out" kids just moved in with you, then you're going to need much more vitamin C. Taking a good source several times a day won't hurt you, especially if you're feeling under the weather. All of us should be taking extra vitamin C. It's cheap insurance and almost impossible to overdose on.

By the way, twenty years ago our medical community scoffed at the idea that vitamin C helped in so many ways, but now they are the first to prescribe it. Didn't your common sense, twenty years ago, tell you that vitamin C was good for you? *Are you really sure you want to rely totally on the western medical community to take care of your health and future?*

Vitamin D — How would you like to get your RDA of a vitamin without eating anything? Exposing yourself to the sun for thirty minutes a day is all you need to get all the vitamin D that your body requires, assuming that you are eating correctly. Now, I know what you're thinking. The answer is no. Taking all of your clothes off and running around naked does not mean that you only need ten minutes daily! That's another experiment that you can do on your own, though. We don't want to be responsible for scaring your neighbors! There is a layer of cholesterol underneath your skin that is transformed into a premature form of vitamin D with exposure to the sun. This, in turn, is sent to the liver and kidneys (via UPS and your blood) where it is made into a useable form of vitamin D. It stays there, reabsorbs calcium from your blood, then ships the calcium back to your system where it can do its magic.

D is required for the utilization of calcium and phosphorus in your body. It helps prevent muscle and bone weakness, prevents osteoporosis in us older folks, protects against cancers and interacts with other helpful agents to make your system run smoothly. You can find D in egg yolks, alfalfa, milk oatmeal, some fish and vegetables. If you choose to supplement it, you must take it with calcium to get the best use of it. Drink a tall glass of milk daily, if you wish. (Although thirty minutes daily is all that is needed to get the minimum daily adult requirement, an hour a day outside will do you a ton of good in more areas of concern than just Vitamin D, and is recommended by this program.)

Vitamin E — This is the *Aerosmith* of vitamins. It's been around for a long time, but is just now becoming a superstar. We're finding several new benefits of vitamin E and reinforcing others. Since E is a fat-soluble antioxidant, it stays in your system longer and does more good than the water-soluble ones, if for no other reason than having "more at bats" than the antioxidants that get washed out of your system quickly. E hangs around in your cell membranes (which are made up primarily of fat) and nukes any antioxidants that try to exit the cell. Because of this, E can prevent and/or minimize many cancers, retard aging, work well with many other vitamins and protect you against heart disease. It may also assist in the fight against Parkinson's disease, diabetes, and benign breast diseases. This is one of the more important supplements to take because it may be a little more difficult to get what you need from a normal diet and it is so important in protecting your future. Again, alfalfa contains E as do some vegetable oils, beans, nuts, whole grains, dark green leafy vegetables, eggs, kelp, flaxseed and oatmeal.

Vitamin K — K stands for "klot." When you cut yourself, vitamin K aids in the "klotting" of your blood — at least it sounds the same. Besides blood clotting (if phonics is so important in school today, then why isn't phonics spelled with an F?), K helps your body hold onto the calcium that it desperately needs to maintain your bones. Thus we have a potential relationship to osteoporosis, the debilitating deterioration of your bones. It also aids in converting glucose into glycogen allowing it to be stored in the liver. (It should be obvious by this point that a healthy liver is crucial to your good health and any substance that can make your liver's job any easier has got to be an all-star!) Other than your heart and brain, your liver is more important than any other organ residing under your skin. Just about anything you put into your mouth goes through your liver. From aspirin to Zocol, your liver has had to cleanse all of the toxins it encounters. It can only take so much before it starts breaking down. Then you are in real trouble! Take care of your liver! K may also help your immune system and promote longevity. Your main source of vitamin K should come from the friendly little bacteria working hard day and night inside of your intestinal tract making K and other helpful elements. However, since you've spent the last twenty years of your life doing your best to destroy any semblance of a healthy digestive system, we'll name some other sources of vitamin K you can use while you're rebuilding up your platoon of little soldiers. You can find vitamin K in alfalfa, green tea, kelp, soybeans, broccoli and other green leafy vegetables, egg yolk and whole wheat. K, being fat-soluble, can be abused by overdosing over a long period of time. As with any other supplements, moderation is the key.

That takes care of all the vitamins, but certainly not all of the players on your team. Vitamins are extremely important, but not anymore so that the remainder of your teammates we are about to discuss.

Minerals

No minerals? You die. A fairly simple but a true statement. Every living thing on this planet needs minerals to survive. From simple amoebas (as in your next-door neighbor) all the way up that biological ladder, mankind needs minerals to exist, and you need a variety of minerals, **all of them taken in balanced amounts for proper absorption.** As different as they all are, each of them, like vitamins, act as coenzymes. In other words, they assist your body in performing all its functions from energy production to building muscle and bone. **Most ailments in mankind can be traced back to a mineral deficiency of some kind or another, a very profound statement if you think about it. Get all of the minerals you need as often as necessary, in the quantity required, and there is a good chance you can kiss a lot of poor health issues goodbye forever!** That may be a pretty bold statement, but if you understand the importance of proper mineral consumption, then maybe you will see the role they play and make a good effort to ensure they are a part of your life.

All minerals are inorganic. In other words, you must consume them from the food you eat or from supplementation because you cannot manufacture them. Minerals come from the soil that vegetation grows in, from the plants that animals eat, then in turn from the vegetation and/or animals that man eats. (Isn't it nice to be at the top of the food chain!)

If you eat plenty of fresh fruits and vegetables grown from your own organic sources, stay clear of the processed and fast-food trappings of the Western world and lead a relaxed life, you're probably getting most of the minerals that you need. Of course the problem is that such a lifestyle or person doesn't exist! We eat on the run, get our meals out of food machines or from the drive up window, and/or from the prepackaged world of so-called energy bars and candy bars. We drink at bars, gulp soda instead of water and skip eating altogether. Then when we do finally cook that special dinner, the vegetables probably have lost their vitamin value from not being fresh at which time we proceed to cook the crap out of them, washing out anything of value. **Face it, you need to supplement your diet with minerals.** Even if you eat better, find fresher foods and cook your vegetables properly, today's farming techniques that stress quantity instead of nutritional quality don't supply the minerals that you need. Our farmlands have been worked too hard depleting them of many of the nutrients needed in the final product. Supplementing vitamins and minerals are easy. You can probably do that with a few capsules daily.

Minerals can be broken down into two basic categories: major and trace. It's pretty simple. You need a lot of calcium, sodium and potassium on a regular basis measured by the gram. The majority of minerals, however, are needed on a much smaller basis. Trace minerals are certainly needed daily, but in much lesser amounts. Some example are: selenium, zinc, chromium and iron. They are all important and can be consumed by having good eating habits and supplementation. Let's briefly discuss the major minerals.

Calcium

Calcium is, by far, the most abundant mineral in your body. You already know that this mineral is important to build strong bones and teeth, but maybe you didn't realize that it does a whole lot more. **Calcium aids the transmission of nerve impulses throughout your body, helps to lower your cholesterol, is necessary for your muscle contractions and helps your blood to clot.** Can it prevent cancer, lower blood pressure and prevent osteoporosis? You bet! **Calcium also maintains the fluid level within each and every cell and activates several important enzymes used in fat metabolism.** Without it your joints would ache, your blood pressure may rise, you could develop arthritis, depression, convulsions and insomnia, among other ailments. Again, just minor little inconveniences.

You can find calcium in dairy products, green vegetables, seafood, brewers yeast, nuts, beans, soybeans, yogurt, alfalfa, kelp, chamomile, flaxseed, parsley, peppermint and many other foods and herbs. An 8-ounce serving of yogurt alone has over 400 milligrams of calcium, approximately a third of your minimum daily requirement. Most multivitamin and mineral supplements will also have calcium included. If you happen to be of the female persuasion, then you already know that this mineral is crucial in your fight against osteoporosis and should not be ignored as an additional supplement even if you eat many of the foods containing calcium. Remember, your system is constantly adjusting the amount of calcium in your blood (primarily to raise the pH level) and requires a constant supply, or it will be forced to remove some from your bones.

Iron

Iron is the mineral of choice of your blood. It aids in the production of hemoglobin and the oxygenation of your red blood cells. Iron also plays a role in nourishing your muscle tissues It is essential to many enzyme processes, assists in energy production and is required to maintain a healthy immune system.

You can become iron deficient from excessive bleeding whether it is external or internal bleeding, long-term illnesses, excessive coffee consumption, ulcers and poor digestion among other things. Signs of a deficiency include: fatigue, hair loss, obesity, dizziness, digestion problems, abnormal-shaped nails and slow mental responsiveness. (That sounds like a bad hangover!) Since iron is stored in your body (fat soluble), excessive buildups can cause problems, many of which have gotten a bad rap recently. There may be an occasional need for iron supplementation, but when you begin eating properly you will probably not need any additional iron unless you have had any of the above-mentioned ailments.

Other than in your garage, iron can be found in the following: alfalfa, almonds, avocados, beans, brewer's yeast (another rich source of many vitamins and minerals), eggs, cayenne, cereals, chamomile, enriched breads, fish, kelp, kidney beans, lentils, paprika, parsley, peppermint, rose hips, sesame seeds soybeans, whole grains and, of course, green leafy vegetables including spinach. As you can see, it is easy to get sufficient levels of iron and is not worth the risks unless you have been diagnosed with a deficiency. A side note: bacteria needs iron to grow in, so don't give it an excuse to flourish if you have already have a bacterial infection by taking iron supplements.

Magnesium

Many cardiac arrests would probably be prevented if a deficiency in magnesium did not exist. This all-important mineral protects your arterial linings from sudden blood pressure changes, cardiac arrhythmia and hypertension. It is vital as a catalyst in energy production and assists in calcium and potassium absorption. It also helps the conductivity of muscle and nerve transmissions, and may assist dissolving kidney stones.

Magnesium protects against asthma, chronic fatigue, depression, insomnia and certain types of cancer. Poor digestion, seizures, irritability, rapid heartbeat and insomnia are all signs of a magnesium deficiency. If you drink heavily, suffer from diarrhea or use diuretics, more magnesium is needed.

Most mineral supplements contain magnesium, but you can get a lot of what you need from many of the same foods and herbs we have been discussing. Apples, avocados, alfalfa, cayenne, chamomile, bananas, fish, meat, dairy products, brown rice, brewer's yeast, garlic, green leafy vegetables and soybeans are many of the sources. Magnesium, which is balanced against calcium in your blood, is a critical mineral needed in your body that a fast-food diet won't satisfy.

Potassium

It has been said that potassium is to soft tissues as calcium is to bones. Keeping your muscles, blood vessels, ligaments and tendons pliable is partially the job of potassium, whose importance has been erroneously diminished as of late. Do not underestimate the importance of this mineral as you grow older. Not only is it important to your soft tissues, it plays a vital role in keeping your nervous system and the rhythm of your heart in balance. It can prevent strokes, is needed for hormonal secretions, can prevent constipation, depression, edema (water retention), insomnia, muscular fatigue, nausea and a glucose intolerance.

It works with sodium to control the water levels both inside and outside of your cells (thus preventing edema), it acts as an antioxidant and works to flush poisons out of your system. As you age, your ability to absorb potassium diminishes so it is imperative that you get enough through a good diet consisting of bananas, melons, yogurt, many other fruits and vegetables, fish, whole grains, brown rice, garlic, wheat bran, sage, red clover and dates. Don't forget organic apple cider vinegar, nature's natural tonic. Put a couple of tablespoons in a cup of hot water, add some honey (which also contains potassium) and drink as a tea before retiring. You will sleep better too!

Other minor minerals

In the name of expedience, we'll buzz through some of the other minerals necessary for proper bodily functions. **Remember that you are from this earth, dirt, and all minerals are necessary in some degree or another.**

Chromium helps maintain your body's tolerance to glucose, which in turn controls the insulin produced by your pancreas. You remember diabetes don't you? With all the sugar we Americans have been cramming down our collective throats all of these years, chromium becomes more important to watch out for.

Copper helps your body absorb iron, acts as an enzyme in the formation of hemoglobin and collagen (a protein found in your skin and tendons) and neutralizes free radicals. (In fact, copper was responsible for rounding up Bobby Seale in the 60s.)

Manganese, not to be confused with magnesium, assists bone and connective tissue growth and activates many enzymes that regulate metabolism. It helps your nerves, immune system, and blood sugar levels. Your joints are lubricated thanks to manganese, which works tirelessly in unison with vitamins E and the Bs without ever asking for more money or paid vacations.

Molybdenum. Who's that? Forget it; just eat correctly!

Phosphorus. Forget him, too. As much soda as you have consumed since Jimmy Carter was president, you probably glow in the dark because of this mineral. On top of that, there is a balance of calcium and phosphorus maintained in your blood. By consuming too much phosphorus, you change that critical relationship. So, to compensate, your system leaches calcium from your bones (your body's calcium storage tanks) causing osteoporosis. Look for phosphoric acid in sodas — another reason to stay away from them.

Selenium. This is an extremely important antioxidant, combining with vitamin E to knock out oxidizing lipids (fats). It guards your heart and liver, which by itself should make it onto your Christmas list. Most good general vitamin and mineral supplements contain selenium. Selenium is one of the more important minerals. You should go out of your way to get as much of this much-needed element as you can. Many vegetables and some nuts contain this mineral.

Sodium is everywhere, you probably get too much now, but it is still vital for life in general. Since you probably consume enough sodium in a year to cure a couple of tons of beef, you'll need more potassium to balance things out. Learn *not* to reach for the salt-shaker!

Sulfur. There are several different forms of sulfur in your system, and they are now getting a lot of attention as they relate to arthritis and joint problems. Chondroitin and glucosamine are two sulfates that come to mind. Sulfurs has many other important functions including making your body resist foreign bacteria growth and slowing the aging process. When searching for foods containing sulfites, garlic and onions are good choices.

A final note on minerals

In the beginning of mankind, we arose out of the soil, and we all will eventually end up in six feet of it. Call it one of those profound cyclical facts of evolution. Most of the minerals of our soils are there to nourish us. If we don't get them through the foods we eat or the supplements that we take, that trip down to the mortuary will come sooner than we would like. Eat correctly and take mineral supplements. Products containing forty or fifty trace minerals are readily available and should be a part of your daily regime. Alfalfa also contains a ton of them. In fact, many of the other "grasses" will also work. Whatever the source that you choose, make minerals a habit. They are just as, if not more important, than vitamins!

HERBS

One of the main underlying theories of this holistic approach to medicine is that the human body, if given the chance, will heal itself. Herbs are the epitome of that belief. Webster's Dictionary defines herbs as "an uncle from the state of New Jersey." No wait, that's the wrong herb. How about, "a soft stemmed plant without woody tissue that will wither and die each year, sometimes having a pleasant odor." Sounds like some former love interests... Okay, we will concentrate on the "plant type" herbs. Let's see, that includes about 10,000 species . . . *this is really going to be a long book!*

Actually, *only* 1,500 botanicals are sold in the U.S., and we're only going to talk about a very few of the best and/or most popular. Again, this is to be done for a matter of expediency. There will be many others you may want to explore. The references listed in the back will help you get there. If not, any good bookstore will have several general herb guides, but remember to pay attention if it seems that the author has an agenda to push a certain herb. Try and remain objective. Also, the most important thing to remember about herbs is this: The *h* in herbs is silent . . . please.

Warning! Do not skip this section because you think that *all* herbs are voodoo medicine. Like Western-based medicines, herbs may or may not produce positive results and in fact may be dangerous to your health. Being organic doesn't necessarily translate to being safe to consume. **As with *any* medicine or *anything* else, you need to be careful about what you put into your body.** That being said, please note — before you dismiss herbs for your personal use — the following statistics:

1. Nearly 80% of the world's population uses herbs for at least a portion of their healthcare needs.

2. Approximately 25% of the drugs that you use today contain botanicals of some type as their active ingredient.
3. The Chinese have been using herbs for over 5,000 years, more than enough time to cull out the ones that don't work.
4. Many other ancient civilizations used herbs extensively for their medicinal needs including: the Hebrews, Romans, Egyptians, Persians, American Indians and people from Arkansas.
5. Many herbs are already being prescribed by medical doctors including: ginkgo biloba, saw palmetto and valerian root.
6. Approximately 15% of all hospital patients experience adverse reactions to prescribed medications, the vast majority of them being of the chemical type and not herbs.
7. In 1994 alone, 104,000 hospital patients died from these prescriptions.
8. There is a bacteria called enterococci that is pretty easily treated with the drug vancomycin. In 1988, certain strains of this bacteria that were resistant to vancomycin (called VRE) appeared in a New York City hospital, and as you can imagine, has spread tremendously. In fact, cases of VRE increased twenty fold from 1989 to 1993, and the bacteria is now found in most countries around the world. Why are we talking about this? 98 percent of all cases of enterococci are contracted inside of a hospital! Since there is no known cure for the VRE strains, almost 100 percent of them are fatal. You may enter a hospital for some disorder, but then come out in worse shape that when you went in! Makes a lot of sense, doesn't it? Moral of the story: Keep your immune system up, stay healthy, stay away from drugs that can compromise your immune system and stay out of hospitals! Herbs will help you accomplish that goal.
9. Walt Disney was afraid of mice . . . Just thought you would like to know that.

Anything that you put into your body has the potential to be dangerous or even fatal, including prescription drugs, over the counter drugs, herbs and your mother-in-law's meatloaf. Being careful should be prudent advice for all of the above, especially the ones that are unregulated like herbs, supplements and that meatloaf. That certainly doesn't exempt the pharmaceuticals. Read the several pages of disclosures and possible side effects included with any print ad for a certain drug and you'll hesitate before putting a chemical in your system that may cause dizziness, nausea, vomiting, seizures, blindness, headaches, depression, arrhythmia, ringing in the ears, erectile problems, ugliness, bad taste and credit problems, among countless other serious reactions!

Herbs get a "bad rap" for several reasons. The lack of regulation in that particular industry and several "bad apples" has spoiled the reputation of many of the beneficial products available. Second, the method that herbs use to work is seldom immediate, so it is difficult to gauge their effectiveness. Remember, they work *with* your system to bring balance so that your system can correct itself. Herbs don't want the limelight or the credit. You may take ginkgo biloba for thirty years and never feel much of anything. The fact that you didn't get Alzheimer's during that period of time may be the only proof that it had some value and was worth the time, money and effort. Most herbs are subtle by nature, and only assist your body in doing its job.

The third reason for the "bad rap" lies in the almighty dollar. Take St. John's wort for depression and there are several multi-billion dollar conglomerates that won't be very happy. They will do their best to prove the ineffectiveness of any approach that jeopardizes their bottom line. Never mind that many, many drugs today originated from a botanical source, but guess what? A plant can't be patented and thus can't be profitable, so their answer is to create the same kind of curative powers from a chemical that they can protect through the patent process and turn into profits. It's just part of the business world and we need to respect that fact. Pharmaceuticals, like any other business are there to make money. However, discount any research or study done criticizing any botanical treatment that has been funded by a pharmaceutical company with something to gain by that report. Unfortunately, many of the studies done today fit into that category.

Case in point is a study funded by the company that markets the most popular anti-depressant drug in the world. The study found St. John's wort ineffective in treating depression. This herb has been prescribed in Europe for many years and has been shown to be effective in many *mild* cases of depression. It may not work for you, but that's not the point. Any study done needs to be as objective as possible to be accurate, and one coming from a company with something to gain by a negative finding should be examined very carefully or discarded in favor of other more objective studies. Besides, if it works only 20% of the time, wouldn't you like to be one of them? St. John's wort is a whole lot less expensive and has a whole lot fewer side effects than just about any of the prescription drugs used for depression. The last reason for herb's bad rap is that if your system is not very effective in processing any the nutrients that you feed it, then it's tough to gauge how any herb is going to work given that inefficiency. In other words, if the food train doesn't stop in your stomach and small intestine long enough to do any good, then anything swallowed will be markedly inefficient. The only way to have efficiency in your digestive system is for that system to be healthy. The way to obtain good digestive health is to follow this program. By the way, the above mentioned study on St. John's wort lasted only six weeks; certainly not long enough to correctly measure the effectiveness of any herb, but gave the company what it needed.

Remember those theories about how man has arrived at this place in time? He has used the plants provided him to feed and nourish him. Herbs do just that. They contain most of the nutrients man needs to survive and flourish.

The following is a *very* short list of some of the better, or more popular herbs available today. Some have a wide variety of uses, some are fairly narrow in their scope of usefulness, and at least two of them should be avoided at any cost. Most of them are fairly inexpensive and none of them should be taken by the cupful. Again, moderation is the key. Take it slowly and give them a chance to work.

Alfalfa

You might have guessed by now that this is one of my favorite herbs. It has been revered by the ancient Arabs, who considered it the "father of all foods" and has been used for everything from kidney stones to fluid retention. Not only does it contain most every vitamin and mineral that you need, it serves two other purposes. One, it helps make you regular. Oh, hallelujah! Let's not under-emphasize that benefit! If perhaps you suffer from allergies, alfalfa can also help to desensitize your system to many of the grasses that set you off. Take some local grown honey with the alfalfa and kiss many of your allergies goodbye. Considered a legume, alfalfa contains eight essential amino acids, most vitamins known to man, many minerals, carotene, an anti-fungus agent and the proverbial kitchen sink of nutrients. Yes, this is one that you should take. The tablets taste like . . . alfalfa, so they aren't the most appetizing of pills to swallow, but take these a couple of times a day. You will notice a difference with this one. Pick one that comes in a coated caplet and it will go down much easier. Note: Many of the other grasses also contain a multitude of nutrients.

Aloe Vera

Aloe, long used for minor skin problems including wound treatments, skin rashes, eczema, dandruff and acne, also has been shown to stimulate the production of disease-fighting white blood cells, which may play a role in the fight against cancer. It is also a mild laxative. Keep an aloe plant in your home for use on your skin. Buy lotions with aloe and you can even occasionally drink the juice as a tonic.

Cayenne Pepper

Hot, hot, hot! Hot is good, especially when treating arthritis and other joint ailments, improving blood circulation and warding off colds and sinus infections. It's good for the heart, kidneys, lungs, pancreas and believe it or not, the stomach. It jump-starts enzyme reactions and aids other herbs and vitamins in your system. Cayenne is easy to cook with. Use it in beans, salads, sauces, drinks and cereal. (Maybe not a good idea on that last one.)

Chamomile

Good for your tummy! This multifaceted herb not only is packed with many vitamins and minerals, it does much more than soothe your poor aching stomach. It's a digestive aid, diuretic, settles your mind and helps you sleep. It's also an anti-inflammatory and can kill a headache. This is a fine tasting nighttime tea especially if you add a touch of honey to the brew.

Cinnamon

This palatable herb seems to have a positive affect on blood sugar level along with stimulating circulation and the flow of energy to your abdominal area. Thus it is beneficial for digestive problems of all kinds. It is also an ingredient of mouthwashes because of its germicidal tendencies. Because of its influence on your blood sugar level (diabetes), make cinnamon a part of your daily regime. Put it in coffee, tea, smoothies, cereals and other baked or fresh foods. In fact, if you make your own coffee in the morning, put some in with the grinds before brewing and a flavorful benefit will be added to your day.

Cranberry

One of the few herbs that has a quick response time. If you have a urinary tract infection, it will kill it virtually overnight!

Also, since it is of a deep color, it contains compounds that keep you healthy. The store-bought juices have more sugar (via other juices) in them than anything else. If you have a problem, use the capsules. If you can find cranberry juice that has a higher concentration of the actual cranberry juice, (at least 25%) then buy it.

Echinecea

Echinecea is the "poster child" of herbs. It not only stimulates your body's natural immune system to fight colds and the flu, but it also has very little side effects, if any. You couldn't ask for a better representative of the family of herbs than this all-star. A member of the sunflower family, echinecea helps increase the production of disease fighting white blood cells and nourishes your lymphatic system. Discovered by the American Indian, it was later adopted for its medicinal qualities by our settlers (probably before they slaughtered the majority of their hosts) and was later dropped from use with the introduction of pharmaceutical medicines and antibiotics. It has made a comeback as of recent, especially in Europe where it is use extensively for its healing qualities. Don't use it all the time, but only when you feel at risk of getting ill, and then often until the symptoms subside.

Feverfew

It has been misnamed. It should be called "Headache-away." Take this herb at the onset of a headache and you might be surprised at the results that you get. Feverfew, Latin for "driver out of fevers" can also do exactly that. It relaxes the blood vessels in your brain and inhibits the secretion of substances that can cause pain or inflammation. Take this for the above, plus arthritis, menstrual pains, muscle tensions and to stimulate your appetite, if needed.

Flax

This seed is an essential fatty acid that was discussed in the chapter on foods and should be a part of your life especially if you don't eat cold-water fish several times a week (very few of us do). It is also good for your bones, nails, teeth and your skin. Even though it is actually a fat, it may play a role in regulating your weight. It can be purchased as a liquid-filled capsule or by the seed. Flax seed must be ground up to be of any benefit, or the seeds will just pass through your system undigested. The ground up seeds will spoil quickly, so buy them in bulk and grind in a coffee grinder as needed, or purchase them already ground up and keep them refrigerated. They are very tasty in salads and soups. This is a must if you don't get sufficient amounts of the fish mentioned above. Flax to the max.

Garlic

Even though garlic was also mentioned in our chapter on food, it should be discussed again since it is such a wonderful plant. The regular use of garlic can lower cholesterol and blood pressure, stimulate your immune system, fight cancer and infection and has the ability to knock out a cold or the flu. It reduces congestion and helps with bronchitis. Garlic contains many sulfur compounds and several other essential minerals that are used in the many applications within your body. We could spend hours discussing the many attributes of garlic (there are many books and articles on the subject), but rest assured that it is one of the best herbs or foods that you can put into your system to combat aging and disease. Peel several bulbs, put them through a food processor and store in your fridge for later use. Use it in salads, soups, casseroles, stews, cereal (just kidding again) and any other dishes that seem appropriate. Whole garlic also can be worn around your neck when your in-laws visit to further enhance your health and that of the people around you!

Ginger

Miss Ginger, made famous on *Gunsmoke,* is also a great anti-nausea herb used for everything from motion sickness to morning sickness. (I know she made me feel better!) But her talents don't stop there. Ginger can be used to treat pain, stiffness and swelling problems. Dizziness and vertigo may even be eliminated by using her talents. When's the last time that you cleansed your colon? That's what I thought. Have some ginger tea over several days and you can leave the roto-router in the garage! This herb will most likely find its way into your system through teas or capsules. Not many recipes call for ginger as part of their ingredients.

Gingko Biloba

A distant relative to Bilbo Baggins, of *The Hobbit* fame, this very old herb has finally made its way into mainstream medicine. Doctors, now routinely prescribe gingko to their Alzheimer's patients to help improve their memory. Unfortunately, by then it's too late because they cannot remember to take their capsules, among other things! By that time, too much damage has been done-so begin taking this now.

The gingko tree, one of the oldest trees in existence, was almost wiped out by the ice age. (The same fate as eight-track tapes and Milton Berle.) Each tree can live to be a thousand years old, not unlike like your mother-in-law, and has many medicinal values dating back to Chinese monks thousands of years ago. Gingko improves blood circulation and vascular integrity to your brain, heart and limbs. It can treat headaches, tinnitus, leg cramps, asthma and kidney disorders.

As old as gingko is, that should be a clue that maybe there is something to this herb and it may be worthwhile to take this on a regular basis. Just begin the habit before you forget to take your pills!

Ginseng

The love potion! Yeah, right. We all know that Viagra is *now* the "love potion." Ginseng, another very old herb has an even longer and more complex history than most any plant ever. The ginseng plant is used to increase stamina, strength, improve blood pressure, regulate diabetes and reduce mental confusion. It is also good to use if you have frequent colds and flu. There are subtle differences between the Asian, American and Siberian versions of this wonderful plant and you should do some research on all three before deciding which one is best for you. Again, we could spend an entire book on the subject of ginseng, but we don't have the time. This is certainly a worthy herb and deserving of further research.

Kava Kava

This herb is so good that you have to say it twice! The root of this endangered low-lying plant is used to promote physical and mental relaxation. It's helpful for depression, insomnia, stress and anxiety. You can find this in many concoctions used to help you sleep better.

Ma Huang (Ephedra)

We'll be quick with this one. Stay away from this or any product that contains any amount of this ingredient unless you don't care about the possibility of having heart damage or even a heart attack. Your drug days are long gone. This is no different than speed. It revs you up and can put incredible strain on your body in general. It may shatter your immune system and then drop you like a cheap date. Ma Huang contains an alkaloid substance called ephedrine (stay away from this one also) that can stimulate you much like an amphetamine. It won't cause you to lose weight, the energy burst will be short-lived and the payback will always be severe. Ephedra is killing young and fit, body-building men; so what do you think it will do to you? Just (don't) do it.

Peppermint

Peppermint has long been used for stomach ailments such as intestinal cramps, bloating from excessive gas, indigestion, and nausea. It can even be used on infants with colic. One of its main ingredients is menthol, which gives peppermint its analgesic effects. It is also mildly antiseptic and is used in mouthwashes and as a cleaning agent. Peppermint teas are easy to fix and are very flavorful.

St. John's Wort

Poor guy. First, he has one of the worst names ever given. Like we want to put something in our system that is called "wort"! Then, since it's mildly effective to treat depression, the pharmaceutical companies are out to "hang it high." This little perennial, meadow plant with bright yellow flowers has been around for a long time. Nobody really knows why it was given its name. Whether it was because it blooms sometime around St. John's Day (June 24) or whether it was his favorite plant (wort is old English for "plant"). Regardless, it has many uses besides treating mild depression. It is a mild anti-inflammatory and can be used for sprains, strains and other swelling. It can help to inhibit viral infections such as herpes, but its main focus today is how it is used to treat anxiety, tension and mild depression. Visit a doctor if you have huge recurring problems on the mental front. Don't try to self-medicate. If you're just feeling down, however, go ahead and give it a try. That is after you have made the life-altering changes laid out in this book first. The dietary, fitness and sleep changes that you make may be enough to take care of any minor chemical imbalances in your system.

One note about St John's wort: If you are going under the effects of a general anesthesia, stop all uses of this herb (to be on the safe side, all herbs) at least a week before the procedure.

Apparently it can alter the effects of many different drugs used during the process of putting you under. Your doctor won't touch you if he knows that you have been on this herb recently.

Saw Palmetto

This small Florida palm tree is man's best friend. Literally. Not women, but for men only. This is the one thing that we men get to claim for ourselves. Women, stay away from our saw palmetto. It's ours. (Us men have to have something that we call our own.) This little herb will promote prostate health, and since women don't have one, it will do them no good. Men, unless you like sharp, cold instruments stuck up your address, then begin taking this herb. Enough said.

Valerian Root

This foul-smelling plant (better just use the capsules) is best known for its treatment relating to insomnia. It relieves anxiety, nervousness and can relax your restless mind and body muscles too. In fact, it can be used for muscle cramps, pain and tension. Like many other herbs, Valerian also improves circulation, which is good for high blood pressure and fatigue. Good to take at night if you are having trouble sleeping.

Again, we could spend the entire book (or books!) on herbs, but we must move on. The final area that we'll discuss will be a hodgepodge of different substances lumped together for simplicity purposes that will bring this chapter on supplements to a close. Supplements are extremely important, unless you have a perfect diet and grow your own organic fruits and vegetables. I didn't think so . . .

One final note on herbs. As in foods and many other substances, overcooking them ruins the nutritional and medicinal value of the plant. If heat is required in the preparation of the plant, use as little as possible for as short of time as you can for the best results.

"OTHERS"

Some of the other substances that don't fit under one of the above classifications are now listed and discussed below. Again, there are many, many other items available for your use and benefit. Do some research and find out what works and what doesn't.

Melatonin

Since we just discussed valerian root, we'll cover melatonin, which has some similar uses. While I don't recommend taking very many hormones, melatonin is one of the exceptions. Hormones are manufactured by your body in one of your endocrine glands (thyroid gland being an example) and make chemical messages that regulate hundreds of functions in your system. Most medical experts recommend not messing with hormones in general, as it can be dangerous to your health. Melatonin is manufactured in a small gland inside your brain called the pineal gland. This, of course, tells your body to go to sleep. Unfortunately, as we age we no longer make as much melatonin as we need. Use this if you have a chronic sleep problem only, not if your sleep problem is only on occasion. Taking this hormone a couple of hours before bedtime for us insomniacs seems to pose less of a risk than the lack of good, consistent and restful sleep does. We have previously discussed the long-term ramifications of poor sleep and taking melatonin may help. If you also have trouble staying asleep once you finally get there, then a combination time release/immediate release tablet may help. They usually contain 1 ½ mg. of each. Also try it to minimize the effects of jet lag.

Glucosamine, Chondroitin, and MSM

These three, taken together, can relieve the pain and help rebuild the cartilage in arthritic areas of your poor, fifty-something, broken down body. These are types of sulfurs, which your body needs. Glucosamine sulfate is an amino sugar naturally formed in your body from glucose, which is used in the formation of cartilage, among other things. Chondroitin sulfate is found in cartilage, tendons and ligaments and is also used in the manufacturing of those cartilage that cap your bone ends. Chondroitin is thought to relieve the pain of osteoarthritis and the repair of the damaged cartilage. MSM is also a necessary sulfur and this type is highly absorbable in your body. The three together seem to work best.

CoQ10

He was an assistant to "Q" in the James Bond movies and was injured after Bond fooled around with one of Q's new weapons and is now on complete disability. Actually, CoQ10 is found throughout your system in the mitochondria, which is the energy producing part of the cells in your body. 95% of all energy produced in your body happens here and none of it can take place without CoQ10. Because your heart works all the time, it is one of the biggest users of this essential compound. Consequently, taking this supplement can go a long way in promoting good health of your respiratory and circulatory systems. It can also aid in reducing blood pressure, is an extra antioxidant and is crucial for the production of energy. This is one of those supplements that may be better for you than you'll realize. It is fat-soluble and best taken with one.

5-HTP

This is an amino acid found in one of the steps of manufacturing serotonin, which is one of the most important chemicals in your brain. Serotonin is important in sleep, relaxation, depression, migraines and tension headaches, fibromyalgia, PMS and obesity. Note: There is an interesting example of the importance of serotonin to your system. The only purpose of one of the most popular drug on the market today to treat depression is that it keeps the levels of serotonin in your brain from breaking down. It just extends the usefulness of serotonin. It doesn't do much else, yet is one of the most successful antidepressants on the market today. As we age, serotonin isn't as plentiful as it used to be and anything that can help increase those levels can be of benefit. (Note; exercising produces serotonin also, but that's too much work. Let's circumvent the process your body already has built into it and just take side effect causing drugs...doesn't make a lot of sense, does it?)

Grape Seed Extract

Grape seed extract is an excellent source of plant flavonoids called PCOs. These flavonoids are a powerful antioxidant and in fact are up to fifty times as potent as beta carotine in searching out and destroying free radicals. The more help that you can get promoting your immune system, the better off you are. These aren't very expensive and are easy to take. Grape seed extract is a must.

Lecithin

This very inexpensive substance, which is found mainly in high-cholesterol, high-fat foods contains a compound called choline. Choline, a phospholipid, is important in the production of acetylcholine, which in turn helps to transmit nerve impulses through communicators called synapses. This biological gobbledy-gook is especially important in your brain. The more efficient this activity is, the better equipped your system will be to fight off memory loss and the symptoms of Alzheimer's disease, two very distinct problems with the aging process. The best usable source of this choline is through your bloodstream and taking lecithin daily increases the levels of choline in your blood, making it more readily available. Unfortunately, getting it from food can be counterproductive to your health because of the usual sources of this important brain builder. That's why it's better to get it through supplementation like granules that can be sprinkled over foods or blended into a drink. Lecithin also plays an important role in blood circulation, the lowering of your cholesterol and enhancing the function of your liver. You haven't heard much about lecithin lately; probably because it is so inexpensive, has been around for a long time, and cannot be patented by a pharmaceutical company looking for profits. That doesn't diminish the importance of this great addition to your diet. A certain "must" in your search for good health as you get older. Purchase it fresh and in capsule form. Take a couple of times daily using the capsules when you can't make use of it fresh.

Acetyl-L-Carnitine and Alpha Lipoic Acid

An extremely important amino acid that assists in transporting fatty acids into your cell's mitochondria for the purpose of producing energy, aceyty-l-carnitine also fights deterioration within the cell. Thus, it has some benefit in your war with Father Time. However, it should be combined with alpha lipoic acid for optimum antioxidant affect.

Alpha lipoic acid is one of the superstars on your antioxidant team because it is water- *and* fat-soluble. That means that instead of being washed out of your system too quickly, it is absorb into your cells for a longer useable life. On top of that, after being broken down into dihydrolipoic acid (DHLA), *this* substance *also* is a viable antioxidant! Alpha lipoic acid's structure is so small that it easily slips in and out of your cell's membranes, which may be one of the reasons that it is so useful. ALA is a very busy soldier, which you can read about in several books. For further information, read *Alpha Lipoic Acid, Nature's Ultimate Antioxidant,* by Dr Julian Whitaker.

These two substances taken together are extremely important in your fight to avoid premature death.

Oil of Oregano

This ain't pizza seasoning. The oregano that you are used to isn't really even true oregano. It's probably derived from thyme or marjoram and isn't harvested from the Mediterranean where the real therapeutic oregano grows wild. There is a huge difference. Basically, the oregano that you use for seasoning has little or no medicinal value. The real oil of oregano, a perennial herb in the mint family, has incredible antiviral, antibacterial, antifungal and antiparasitic properties. It stops just about anything that can do damage to you, from toe fungal infections to diarrhea and intestinal worms. It contains a plethora of minerals including: zinc, iron, potassium, calcium and manganese. It will destroy any variety of fungi and yeasts, and it doesn't care where they reside. Have adult acne? Not anymore. Oil of oregano will wipe it out.

This is a great tool in your arsenal against all sorts of age related matters, but you have to make sure that you are getting the pure oil of oregano and not some watered down version. Read *The Cure is in the Cupboard,* by Dr Cass Ingram and your jaw will drop when you learn of this herb's assets. This book is an easy read and will be worth reading. You can purchase the real McCoy from North American Herb and Spice, or my favorite, Survival Enterprises at survival.com.mx/health/oregano. Don't overindulge in this internally. It is such a good antibacterial that it may thin out your beneficial intestinal bacteria if consumed too extensively.

There are countless other valuable substances out there like Conjugated Linoleic Acid, digestive enzymes, natural sweeteners like Stevia root, bee pollen, spirulina, goldenseal, boswellia, milk thistle and the list goes on.

In today's world, supplements *are not* supplemental. They are vital to your health and should be a part of your routine each and every day. As you begin to improve your diet, start new and good habits that will put you on a path to good health and turn to supplements of all types to keep your motor fine-tuned. Begin with a good multi vitamin with minerals, add some of the other substances mentioned here and you will begin to get a sense of the ones that will work best for you. Remember, **you** are the one in charge of **your** health and taking supplements puts you back into the driver's seat.

Step 6:

All My Ex's Live in Texas

(Unfortunately, So Do I) Stress — The Silent Assassin

This murderer is tough to catch. In fact, he's never even been properly identified, much less caught. He's more slippery than *any* terrorist and has killed more Americans than all airplane accidents and wars tallied together. He's probably in your body right now, wrecking all sorts of havoc on your immune, circulatory and digestive systems. And when you get ill, contract some sort of ailment, or in fact die, he'll skip town and never get blamed. Your doctor won't attempt to rid you of, or help you deal with him, and will only prescribe something to ease the symptoms. You occasionally think of him, but figure that he'll just stick around like some unwanted relative. You'll eventually blame everything else on your predicament and never even know what role he actually played . . . until now.

Who is he? We're talking about stress, the so-called "silent killer." He's *back* and playing at a theater nearer to you than you may realize.

What was originally designed to protect man against eminent danger from animals bigger than him has manifested into something else entirely. The stress that we normally think about is actually your body's "fight or flight" response. This has been around since day one of man's existence and we probably wouldn't be here today if he hadn't been able to fight off or run from those saber-toothed tigers and any other prehistoric creatures or problems early man faced. A chilled-out, laid-back, calm response to an attack by a not-too-friendly beast wouldn't be very effective in fighting it off or fleeing the scene. If we didn't have the ability to "get stressed," wild dogs would now be ruling earth, instead of man . . . I mean woman.

When something happens that scares you, your sympathetic nervous system (no, it's not an empathetic and caring nervous system) kicks in, pumping out cortisol and other stress hormones that increase blood pressure, muscle tension and your heart rate. Cortisol's job in this particular instance is to make sure your blood is supercharged and your body is ready to face or run from whatever is attacking you, like Girl Scouts selling cookies. It pumps glucose, fatty and amino acids out of your tissues and into your blood circulation with the idea of turning you into Superman or Wonder Woman, at least for that moment. (This is a perfect example of the theory "survival of the fittest." Only the humans that could produce this response survived to the next set of generations and the genetic material needed to replicate this response was imbedded into future generations of man.)

Fast forward now to present day metropolis. It's okay and necessary for this response to happen occasionally, Lord only knows we have enough Girl Scout cookies in our pantries to feed several third-world countries. The problem arises when your stress hormone levels stay active for too long and too often. In other words, it wasn't designed for people that are uptight and stressed all the time. This activity was designed only for actual emergencies and can do some real damage in the long run if called upon too often. If you are constantly signaling for this response, your body is never able to store the necessary hormones needed and this increases the risk of many metabolic disorders. It's like crying wolf internally. The same thing applies to your car. If you filled your automobile with nitro or another supercharger and then constantly revved your engine, you'd be buying a new car much sooner than desired. Those type of superchargers are meant for only occasional use. Too much use of superchargers burns out your engine...the same holds true with your body and its relation to stress.

RESULTS OF STRESS

There is a huge array of problems associated with chronic stress. All of them are potentially life threatening, and controlling your exposure to this monster cannot be emphasized enough.

When your cortisol level remains high, your body is encouraged to store fat, probably since fat is mainly where cortisol is kept. To make matters worse, for some reason it is usually stored around your belly. (Look at yourself and deduce where your excess fat is. If you have the proverbial beer gut, then the stress in your life may be contributing to your waistline!) On top of that, studies have shown that people with higher stress-induced cortisol levels tend to eat more. Obviously, we know where this point is headed. Also, related to this, higher than normal insulin levels occur with excess cortisol in your bloodstream, which can make your body less responsive to insulin. **If continued long enough, this can lead to diabetes, something no one wants. Contract diabetes and you better have good life insurance.**

Dumb and Dumber

Have trouble thinking when you're stressed? There are actually biological reasons for this problem . . . It is not just you. Researchers believe that chronic stress can damage a part of your brain called the hippocampus, which controls learning and memory. When you're constantly stressed, so is your brain. It's harder to think straight when you're preoccupied with whatever is causing you tension. Stress, in general, "trashes" your brain causing other types of problems, many of which may lead to several different nervous system diseases and disorders.

Have a heart

Heart disease and strokes can introduce themselves to you personally because of stress. Under stress, fat is released into your blood system raising blood serum cholesterol. Remember that we need supercharged blood to confront this perceived danger. Your blood pressure rises and unwanted clotting activity begins. Higher levels of homocysteine (a risk factor in artherosclerosis) are also common among the stressed. Angina, which is severe chest pains, is also a warning sign of impending heart disease. It is very common in stressed-out or angry people. All of these lead to higher incidences of heart and other circulatory diseases.

In stressed women, estrogen levels may be reduced, compounding the problem. Low levels of estrogen can lead to menopause and low sexual interest, among other maladies.

People can, and do, die as a direct result of stress-related situations. Now you know why. One of the main goals of this program is to keep you from becoming a statistic and being stressed will earn you your stripes quicker than necessary!

Burp! Excuse me!

Everyone has had heartburn and other digestive problems

before. Emotional well-being is important and is one of the factors in a smooth-running digestion system. Your brain can greatly affect the autonomic nerves that control the flow of food through your entire digestive system. Let's face it, much of your digestive system is nothing more than muscles that massage and contract, processing and moving food along until your system has fully used what it needs and then is ready to flush the remaining waste down that proverbial chute. Disrupt some of those all important brain chemicals and you can have major league problems. "Freeze up" those muscles, and life can get a little uncomfortable. Constipation is something we all have been through that not only can be painful, but, over the long-term, can also be dangerous to your overall health. Chronic constipation leads to several other maladies, discussed previously. Long-term stress only helps to prolong and promote those.

Zit face

Do you remember "getting stressed" and immediately breaking out with some sort of rash, irritation, pimples or canker sores? **Since your skin has so many nerve endings, stress has a habit of finding its way to your body's surface. Rosacea, eczema, hives and psoriasis are some of the ailments "helped along" by chronic stress.** If nothing else, your vanity should step in and give you some more incentive to rid yourself of excess stress. No one wants these ugly problems.

Call me crazy

Almost half of all Americans have or will have depression and/or anxiety-related problems, whether temporary or long-term. **Stress causes and/or exasperates emotional problems** for several reasons. First is the lack of sleep caused by stress. No sleep, no rest. No rest, no hormones and endorphins manufactured in your brain. These particular chemicals are crucial in maintaining the proper chemical balance in your brain, which in turn, contributes to your emotional well being. Stress may not make you crazy by itself, but it sure can help it along.

Ouch

Chronic pain caused by stress adds to the dilemma. The muscle tension associated with emotional discomfort can contribute to TMJ, back and neck pain, headaches and an overall lowering of your pain threshold. Many times stress will manifest itself in the weakest part of your body. If you suffer from chronic pain, getting stressed can cause the pain to be felt there, like in your neck or back. Having constant pain can also make you more susceptible to mental ailments such as depression discussed above. People with fibromyalgia, rheumatoid arthritis and other chronic pain are susceptible to emotional problems, if those ailments bother them for an extended period of time.

Austin Powers

Stay stressed too long and your interest in sex may diminish. Yes, even you. It can, and maybe already has happened to you or your mate. Of course, all you have to do is join the priesthood and your sexual energy will suddenly reappear. If that's not an option, then removing excess unhappiness from your life can reap passionate benefits. Stress is mean and ugly! Uptight men can become impotent (does not mean important), women can have trouble reaching orgasm and also are susceptible to irregular menstrual cycles. It's even been blamed on infertility! Last, but certainly not least, PMS symptoms are intensified under stressful conditions, which as you know, can clear out an entire room of bingo players!

According to the National Institute of Mental Health (I'm

their poster child and honorary lifetime member!), 70-80% of all doctor's visits are for stress-related illnesses! It's not the stress itself, but what really matters is where it rears its ugly head and then how you deal with it.

Today we have stressful jobs, traffic, kids that flat wear us out, difficult marriages, enough financial worries to create a tidal wave of problems . . . insurance, retirement, college costs, medicine's skyrocketing prices, and increasing cost of all sorts of services. Try and take a vacation to get away from all of it, and instead, the exorbitant costs involved in just taking that "restful" vacation can . . . well, you get the point.

ARE YOU STRESSED?

A certain amount of stress is necessary and even beneficial for a normal life. How do you know if what you have is normal or not? Other than obvious signs of how you are feeling, one of the ways to tell is whether you have too many circumstances in your personal environment that may be contributing to your overall level of stress.

The list on page 229 contains many "potential" stress triggers that can influence your level of stress. (**Try and remember that the level of stress is not the circumstance itself, but how you react to it.**) From CEOs, presidents and politicians to housewives, salesmen and teachers, from accountants to zookeepers, many people have a ton of potentially stress-causing situations in their lives; some handle them beautifully and others succumb to the pressures and end up having emotional and physical problems. It doesn't mean that the ones that are the most affected are any less of a person than the others (politicians excluded!), it just indicates that they haven't handled the stuff thrown at them as well as they possibly could have. You are now taking charge of your life and future well being, and this is one of the areas that will demand your utmost attention. It may be one of the most difficult improvements for you to accomplish, but is crucial to your health. Have something tragic happen in your life and yes, stress will happen. That's normal. It's when everyday life keeps you in a constant state of unnecessary readiness for that "fight or flight" response that the problems occur.

You can see, from the list on the opposite page, that many different things add to the big bonfire that can fuel the dilemma of stress. Most are negative in nature, but not always. Anything that adds to your total "load," whether it be of time, commitment, responsibility or just adding to the confusion of that thing we call life, can be stressful. If you aced this test, then chances are that stress is causing all sorts of havoc on your life. Time to whip its butt!

Do you know this person?

Some people seem to thrive on stress as though it is the glue that holds them together. The more that they have, the more they seem to rise to the occasion. They may seem okay . . . now . . . but they're in a pressure cooker and eventually it will catch up to them. When it does it usually causes a pretty steep decline . . . to put it nicely. Crash and burn is more like it. Our tiny little brains can only handle so much. We all need to release the pressure caused by the stresses of everyday life, or better yet, get rid of some of those ankle chains before they drag us down into the pits of Hell. There needs to be some sort of balance. Problems, pressures and stress, in general don't just go away and they usually don't just work themselves into a solution. They all have to be confronted sometime, preferably on your own time. If you take control of your life and decide to tackle them as they appear, or at least learn to live with it, then you'll be much better able to handle life in general, leading to a longer, healthier life.

Here's the list. You probably have, or have had at least some of these situations recently:

1. Death of a spouse. (That would be an understatement!)
2. Divorce. (Sometimes a reduction of stress!)
3. Marital separation.
4. Jail time. (Oops.)
5. Death of a close family member.
6. Personal injury or illness.
7. Marriage.
8. Fired from a job.
9. Marital reconciliation. (Why on earth would you do that?)
10. Retirement. (Now what do you do with your time?)
11. Health change of a family member.
12. Pregnancy. (Oops, again.)
13. Sexual difficulties.
14. Gain a new family member. (Whether you want them or not.)
15. Business readjustment. (Like Wal-mart moving in and putting you out of business.)
16. Change in financial state. (Usually for the worse, but not always.)
17. Death of a close friend.
18. Change in a line of work.
19. Change in number of disputes with spouse.
20. Large mortgage. (Any mortgage, for that matter.)
21. Foreclosure. (Ouch again.)
22. Change in work responsibilities.
23. Child leaves home. (And then, inevitably, they come back.)
24. Outstanding personal achievement. (Positive things also cause stress.)
25. Trouble with the law. (Or trouble with the in-laws, too!)
26. Spouse starts or stops work.
27. Change in living conditions. (As in getting kicked out of your house by your spouse!)
28. Change in working hours.
29. Change in residence. (Moving is big-time stress.)
30. Change in sleeping habits. (Doesn't help matters any.)
31. Change in eating habits.
32. Christmas or Chanukah. (Extremely stressful for many.)
33. Vacations. (Need a vacation from your vacation?)
34. Pet dies. (Sometimes more of a loss than losing a spouse!)

THAT'S EASY FOR YOU TO SAY!

Anyone can tell you that you need to just "deal with your stress." Actually taking care of the stress triggers and making your life simpler is much easier said than done, as we all know. This program cannot even begin to act as an emotional panacea. All that it can possibly do is to help you see what stress is doing to your life and health, possibly steering you in the right direction.

Knowing that too much stress *is*, and *can be,* dangerous to your long-term well being, how do you get rid of it? The simple answer is, concerning at least some of it, you don't. You can't "get rid of" many of the things that add to the level of your stress, but you can learn to manage most of them.

10 WAYS TO REDUCE STRESS

The following is a list of the top-ten ways to quickly reduce stress. Finding ways to reduce or eliminate the pressures in your life cannot be overstated. Hope some of these work for you.

1. Use your MasterCard to pay off your Visa account.
2. When someone says, "have a nice day," tell him or her that you have made other plans.
3. Make a "things to do list" of things you have already done.
4. Forget the diet and send yourself a candy gram.
5. Start a vicious rumor and see if you can recognize it by the time it gets back to you.
6. Write a short story, using alphabet soup.
7. Make up a language and ask people for directions.
8. Paste your mother-in-law's picture on a Playboy centerfold and mail it to her minister.
9. Give your cat a tongue bath.
10. When a telemarketer asks for you, tell them that you have just died and then wait for their reaction.

Wrong list again! This may be fun and they might actually reduce a little bit of stress, but they won't solve most of the real problems we busy Americans have. There are literally hundreds of ways to alleviate and tone down the effects on your mind and body from stress. Since stress is really about the way that you handle both positive and negative circumstances, what works for you may not work for others. However, there are several areas of concern that need to be looked at that will make dealing with stress, in general, much easier. You will also notice that all ten of these promote good health in general and that the solutions are very logical.

The (Real) Top Ten Stress Busters

1. **Exercise.** Countless studies have shown that a regular exercise program greatly assists in reducing stress. Besides providing a release of frustrations, taking your mind off the perils of everyday life, and giving you a sense of accomplishment, exercise releases all kinds of endorphins plus the hormone called serotonin that literally assists in putting your mind at ease. These brain chemicals are extremely important in several different crucial functions, calming your body being one of them. Working out reduces chronic pain, increases the efficiency of your circulatory system, helps you sleep better and drives many toxins out of your system. All of these are major stress reducers. Not only will you feel better about yourself, you will actually be in better physical condition, which is important in fighting any and all problems that you may have, stress being one of them. Let's not forget about how good exercise makes you feel. Stress reduction is another grand reason for beginning a lifelong exercise program.
2. **Diet.** Another one of those areas that help all sorts of different bodily functions. Make sure you're getting enough vitamin C and E, preferably from the food that you eat. Vitamin C is the stress vitamin and protects your system from the ravages of

trauma. The Bs are also important since they cover proper brain and nervous system functioning. When you're feeling stressed, stay away from protein rich foods and concentrate on starchy types of foods like whole wheat breads, fruits and vegetables. The extra carbohydrates that make up the starchy foods help in the release of serotonin, according to Rob Markus, Ph.D. and author of a Dutch study on the subject. Also avoid the junk and any high simple sugar treats that may give you instant gratification, but by spiking your blood sugar level will cause more long-term problems thus contributing to your tension. (Maybe bon-bons aren't such a good idea.) Herbs such as chamomile, valerian root, ginseng and ashwagangha (who?) all have specific uses that may help. Again, "you are what you eat."

You're also "what you drink." David Posen, M.D. and author of *Always Change a Losing Game* said, "Eliminating caffeine is more effective than any other stress-reduction strategy I know." He says that 75% of his patients that cut the caffeine feel much more relaxed and actually have more energy, most likely from the better rest that they are now receiving.

3. **Shut-eye.** Proper rest is paramount in dealing with stress. A strong mind and a strong body give you the defense you need in fighting stress. Sleep is extremely important in both. As mentioned in the chapter devoted to sleep, a good night's rest resets your brain, releases human growth hormones, serotonin and other chemicals necessary in having a sound mind, and generally heals what ails you. Nothing beats a good night's sleep.
4. **Work on your relationships.** By the time you have reached middle-age, you can probably count the number of *good* friends you have on one hand . . . and maybe even have fingers left over! By the time you die, you'll have less. Nothing is better than good friends and family to soothe the soul. If you don't have as many good relationships as you think you should, take

the time and effort to cultivate new ones and them nurture them and the ones you already have. You probably buried yourself in your job, kids and spouse for the last couple of decades. Good, that's where you needed to be. However, now you need some "me" time. At some point your kids will have moved away or will have lost interest in you, the friends you thought you had, aren't, or maybe death will strike closer than you wish. Your spouse could decide that he/she is tired of putting up with you and all of your issues, and then leaves. Then what? You need to have good quality relationships regardless of your current situation. Contact your old high school and college friends. How about former fellow employees that you remember as good people? Seek out friendship in your church. Join the YMCA or take up a hobby that involves interacting with other people. Good relationships with your "support network" cannot be over emphasized enough. Who can you turn to in time of need? What about just a caring voice that will listen to some of your problems? Maintaining good quality friendships can be an effective weapon in fighting stress.

A Michigan study, scheduled to run in *Psychological Science,* demonstrated that older people that gave time, emotional support and energy to friends, family and spouses will more than likely live longer than those simply on the receiving end of kindness. The study done on 423 senior Michigan couples took into account age, sex, health, wealth and many other factors that would affect longevity and found that the people who gave more of themselves tended to live longer, possibly from the emotional lift one gets from helping others.

5. **Spirituality.** Whether or not you believe in Christ, Moses, the Koran, sacred cows or even just yourself, believe . . . in something. You need to believe that there is a reason for being here, if not, then not having a purpose in life becomes a stumbling

block in dealing with stress. You must love yourself before you can love anybody else and to love yourself, knowing that there is a reason for your existence is very important. Spirituality is very important in dealing with disease, trauma, overall health and of course stress. An example of the effects of spirituality on your health was demonstrated by a 1998 Duke University study on churchgoers. They found that people who attended church were healthier, but if they did get sick, they also recovered quicker than the non-attendees.

6. **Massage and other alternative therapies.** Loosening up your tight muscles, getting rid of aches and pains, releasing some hormones and other natural chemicals are all byproducts of getting a massage, having acupuncture, acupressure, or other "touch" type of bodywork done. They can be very beneficial in dealing with the muscle tension and other pressures caused at least indirectly by stress. Also, the actual "touching" itself of your body by another person has benefits too. Although you may be uncomfortable in the beginning, relax and enjoy. In terms of instant gratification as it pertains to stress reduction, massage is right up there with the best.
7. **Take a "chill pill."** In other words, do more of the things that you already find relaxing. If it's golf, knitting, reading, sightseeing or enjoying entertainment, just do more. We never seem to have enough time for ourselves. We're always putting the needs of others in front of ours. That's fine, if there's a specific need of that person. For the most part, we have gotten so used to doing things for other people (like our kids) that we just automatically continue that behavior. **In the long run, you cannot take care of others until you first take care of you.** Go ride a bike or travel more. You deserve it and your body will react in kind.

   Let's put meditation in this category. In its simplest form, meditation is nothing more than a concentrated focus. It gets a bad rap as being more like voodoo than medicine, when in fact, fifteen minutes a day of any forms of this focus is all you need to reduce anxiety, blood pressure, PMS, headaches and coronary arrhythmia. You've got fifteen minutes, don't you? I thought so. Simply focusing on your breath, heartbeat, a mantra (can you say Hari Krishna?) or just relaxing by itself can do wonders for your psyche. The relaxation response is obviously the opposite of the fight-or-flight reaction that we're trying so hard to get rid of and that's why it works so well. The actual physical response is similar to what happens when you take beta-blockers, but without the potential side effects!

8. **You're killing my funny bone! (Have a good laugh.)** The importance of laughter as it pertains to your health and well being is one of the most under-rated and under-utilized tool at your disposal . . . and you don't even have to work for it! The average child laughs or smiles approximately 400 times a day. (Yes, I did count.) By the time that child reaches adulthood the number decreases to fifteen times a day. (Side note: I once went twelve days and only smiled three times! Damn proud of it, too!) What happened between childhood and old fart-hood? Of course, the simple answer is "Life happens." Somewhere along the way you stopped laughing, and that's killing you or at least keeping you from reaching your optimum level of health. All kinds of studies show a correlation between the amount of laughter in one's life and their overall health, especially pertaining to coronary heart disease.

    Dr. Lee Berk, a research doctor at U.C. Irvine says, "Laughter is like taking an internal jog. Your heart rate elevates, blood pressure increases, muscles contract and oxygen levels rise." What a way to get exercise! The American Heart Association presented a study of 300 patients, half with heart disease the other half being healthy. The half with heart disease were 40% less likely to find humor in certain circumstances than the healthy half. That's significant!

Another study showed that heart attack victims were less likely to suffer a second heart attack if they laughed for only thirty minutes a day. That's watching only one congressional news conference a day! Think there's nothing to this? Think again. There are over 300 "laughter clubs" (not comedy clubs) in the U.S. and Canada that, you guessed it, their only purpose is to induce laughter for better health. (They probably show some political speeches! Why? Because they are funny.) Sorry, the question was, "Why are these *clubs* so popular?" Laughter stimulates at least a mild cardiovascular workout. It relaxes muscles and helps fight chronic pain and illnesses. Getting funny actually produces endorphins that stop the production of our friend, Mr. Cortisol.

Another by-product of stress is that it injures the lining of your blood vessels that can lead to a heart attack. Laughter releases nitric oxide (not to be confused with laughing gas) that relaxes your blood vessels, which in turn lessens the occurrence of heart attacks. It also increases the level of a certain antibody that fights bacterial and viral infections of the upper respiratory and gastrointestinal systems. Pretty heady stuff for something that feels so good. So, take your favorite person out and have a nice healthy meal with some red wine and venture into a comedy club afterward. **The happier you are, the more you laugh, and the healthier you will be . . . that's a physiological fact.**

9. **Go light on the sauce.** Alcohol bumps up the production of cortisol. Maybe that's why there are so many angry drunks. The National Heart, Lung and Blood Institute's blood pressure education program says to limit alcohol consumption to two drinks a day. (Skip a couple of days and you don't get to drink the ones you missed!) Enough said on this one. If stress is a problem in your life, then maybe alcohol is too . . .
10. **Last, but certainly not least.** In fact, this is probably one of the more important stress busters. Take control . . . of *your* day,

your life, *your* home, *your* time, *your* money . . . whatever it is that is out of control. Get a handle on it! If you have a job that wears you out physically and emotionally, either figure out a way to smooth out the rough edges or get another one. It's not worth it. In a burdensome relationship? Time to lessen the load. Tell the loser to take a hike. I know, easier said than done. But at some point you have to ask yourself whether it's worth it or not.

Remember, you cannot control *everything*. So, let some things go. If your nineteen year old (the one that's still living at home) doesn't keep his room the way he should, and you have been after him (or her) for years; give it up. You've done *your* part and put in *your* time. He's a man now and is, or will be responsible for himself, so let him make his own mistakes. Maybe he'll learn from them . . . fat chance! The point is that it's not your fight anymore. Can't get everything done each day that you try to do? Just do what you can, giving it your best effort and save the rest for another day.

Also, on the issue of control: **Don't sweat the things that you cannot control** . . . like traffic. There's not a damn thing you can do about a traffic jam. Weaving in and out of traffic may, at best, save you five minutes. It's not worth it! Instead take a great CD, turn up the volume and have a good time. Just remember you don't want the idiots next to you to have as much fun as you so keep your windows rolled up and the air guitar act to a minimum! Tons of books have been written about gaining control of things. Hell, there are several lecture circuits out there that preach nothing but getting control as it pertains to your career, home and children. It would be impossible to touch on all aspects of control here, but just being aware of it and how it can affect your level of stress may be enough to help thing out. **This is worth repeating and stressing (pardon the pun). Don't sweat the things that you cannot control.**

WHEN ALL ELSE FAILS...

There is one last way to look at stress . . . and that is that it doesn't really exist. No, really. Since most of the animals that caused man eminent and physical danger have long become extinct, stress doesn't have any logical or physical root. It is not a disease since there is no virus, bacteria or anything else that can cause an ailment that kills way too many of us each and every year.

A Dr. Hans Selye created this malady in 1936. (Right in the middle of the Great Depression sounds like a good time to have launched this ailment called stress!) It just suddenly appeared. All of the sudden we now had "stress" and didn't have it before? Think about it. Stress is a bundle of symptoms and nothing more. Granted, those symptoms can knock the crap out of you, but what actually caused the symptoms? Cancers have an origin, so does heart disease, the flu, strokes and neurological disorders. All of them can be traced, at least somewhat, to some particular breakdown within your body. What physically defective collapse caused your stress?

Stress is actually nothing more than fear. It is fear of something, someone, some action or a future occurrence. You're not really stressed; you are afraid of something, whether it is a responsibility, a challenge, or maybe your world is falling in around you and in that case the fear of collapse and failure can make your life miserable. According to Dr. Robert Maurer, a clinical psychologist at the UCLA School of Medicine, "There are only two basic fears: One is that you're not worthwhile or good enough to get the job, the recognition, or whatever, and the other is that you are going to lose control, such as in health or financial concerns." All stress can be broken down into one of those two categories. I know mine is based on a lack of control of my life and where it may be headed. There, I feel better already! What's yours?

Kids don't generally have a problem with stress. They call it fear, or being scared. They are not fearful to *say* that they are afraid and neither should you. They don't bury it somewhere and wait for it to rear its ugly face sometime later down the road. They react then and there. Children unconsciously realize that while they don't have much control over their world and have much to fear, it's just a normal part of growing up. Why don't grownups have the same realization?

Recognize stress as nothing more than a fear of something and that it is a normal part of a complex life. In fact, the more complicated your life, the more "stress" there is. The higher up on that totem pole that you go, the more fear there is to face. It's like climbing a ladder. The further you climb, the scarier it can get. Fears are something that we all have to face, sooner or later. Ignoring them or running from them will not solve the situation and it will more than likely show up somewhere else or some other time. Rather, you should face them head-on and approach them as a challenge.

Try to recognize that *fear* is what you are feeling, not *stress.* **Stress doesn't exist in any physical form.** Once you recognize that, (identify the true source of your fear), only then will you be able to work through whatever it is that is bothering you. Face your fears and maybe the stress will go away.

Remember, "stressed" spelled backwards is "desserts" . . . I'm not sure exactly what that means, but I'm sure that you can figure some relevance to it and then make stress a positive experience!

Step 7:

Defensive Driving

When you think of defensive driving, the first thought that comes to mind is to put your hands at ten and two on the steering wheel, keep a safe distance between you and the car in front of you, (which for me is about three feet) and generally be aware of all that is on going around you. Well, we're not talking about ***that*** type of defensive driving. We'll make the assumption that you have mastered those particular skills enough so at least to have kept you alive until now. You may not always use them, but at least you know what they are in case you spot a squad car hiding under a billboard.

The defensive driving covered here has to do more with how you live your life and whether on not you're practicing good "driving" habits on your journey to a long and comfortable life. Are you a conscientious, or reckless driver? Are you doing all that you can to preserve the chances that you will live a long and comfortable life, or at the other end of the spectrum, are you doing all you can to destroy your life and the lives of those around you? Maybe you're just "winging it" day by day with no direction, plan or purpose. Run your ***car*** into the ground and you'll be buying another . . . soon. Unfortunately, you don't have that luxury with your body, although you can buy new kidneys, a liver, or maybe a slightly used heart, none of which are an easy or desirable option, to say the least.

There are some similarities between the care of your body and the type of defensive driving emphasized in high school driving courses. In particular, "generally being aware of all that is going on around you" is an important key to longevity. **You want to do all that you can that will increase your percentages of living a long and happy life.** Drinking and staying out all night several nights a week for the next several years ain't gonna get you there. Neither will smoking cigarettes or even spending a lot of time in a smoke-filled environment. Deciding to take up rock climbing when you're fifty-something and fifty pounds overweight isn't as good of a choice as hiking up steep hills on a regular basis (every bit as stimulating and will do wonders for your health without the threat of a quick and immediate death.) The human body doesn't bounce very well, especially dropped from a rock 200 feet above! At our age, it doesn't react well to even falling on the ground or pavement from no higher up than the standing position, let alone from a rock ledge.

You already know many of the obvious ways to damage or kill yourself: drinking way too much way too often, living on a diet of donuts and ding dongs, burning that proverbial candle at both ends and/or living on the edge, in general.

The Homo sapiens that dwell on this North American continent (that would be we Americans) all seem to all live by the credo that states "**What you can't see, won't hurt you.**" **Unfortunately, most of the "things" that *can* and *will* hurt you cannot be seen by the naked eye.** All the little varmints like bacteria, viruses, ultraviolet rays, poisoning from inorganic minerals, radon, molds, parasites, and the IRS can all make your life miserable if not end it entirely. Most allergy attacks, cases of food poisoning and the flu, chronic fatigue, arthritic symptoms, and a whole array of other ailments can all be attributed to "things" you cannot see, many of which can be controlled. Breathe the wrong air long enough and you can end up in a wheelchair. Not taking the proper steps to strengthen your immune system and you're liable to catch everything that comes along, further weakening your defenses. Not having a "healthy" respect for the parts of Mother Nature that can cause damage and you can bet that she will take out her wrath on you. **We're not worried about arrows and bullets; we're concerned about microbes and molds.**

LITTLE PINK HOUSES

Mi casa es su casa. Let's start as close to home as possible . . . like where you live. We think of our home as our safe haven, our protection from the cruel, mean, cold world. It's our refuge, our oasis, our comfort zone, and it may be killing us. Maybe a slight overstatement, but not entirely so. One example of a possible danger lurking in your home has to do with your gas furnace, if you have one. If it is old, especially if it is has a pilot light and not ignition fired (like a spark plug in your car), there is a definite chance that the heat exchanger has a crack in it. It is a nature of the beast, so to speak, and happens quite frequently, even if it's a newer unit. **If it is cracked, it is letting carbon monoxide** (a **poisonous gas) into your home, which can make you ill, if not put you to sleep and then kill you.** (You cannot smell carbon monoxide, either.) Heat exchangers cannot be repaired, so they need to be replaced now. Also, if the pilot light is out in your furnace or even your water heaters, they are venting gas into your home. If that is the case, you can probably smell that. Natural gas, in its original form, has no odor, but your friendly gas company puts some in to protect you. (This leaking of any type of household gas is obviously dangerous, too.) Have your HVAC system checked and cleaned on a regular basis, probably twice a year as you are going into the fall and spring. You may want to think about installing a carbon monoxide detector as another check. They run about $20–40 and could give you peace of mind. There have been many cases of people living with the above scenarios for years, suffering many debilitating disorders and never having a clue of why they were sick.

Do you have carpeting? If so, how old is it? Was it installed during the Kennedy administration? Do you have indoor/outdoor pets? (Homes that have all hardwood, vinyl, or tile floors will probably not have the following problems.) Do you treat your yard for insects? If yes to the above, you'll be surprised to read the following. Studies have shown that families with indoor/outdoor pets have up to 50 times the levels of diazinon (an insecticide) in the air and carpeting ***inside*** their homes as compared to outside within their yards! The reason why is that pets and people, mainly kids, track the poison in from their yard and over time the residue builds up. Since your home is a closed environment, the poisons have nowhere to go. They cannot be flushed away into your sewer system, eventually coming back to you through your drinking water. The insecticide just stays right there in your carpeting. Your overall exposure to chemical poisons, including most commercial insecticides has never been greater.

These insecticides work by disrupting and breaking down the nervous systems of the insects targeted and unfortunately mammals, like man, rely on the same type of neurotransmitters as the bugs do. The results we are seeing is that the ever increasing numbers of neurological disorders such as Parkinson's, Alzheimer's, and ALS (Lou Gehrig's Disease) could very well be enhanced as a result of your exposure to these poisons. These disorders are at epidemic proportions, which correlate very nicely with our increased usage of these insecticides. It has been noted that agricultural communities using a lot of insecticides show a higher level of these diseases than non-ag areas. Also, people who work in those particular industries have been shown to have a higher risk of contracting these maladies. Merely coincidence? Are you willing to bet your health on it? I didn't think so. To compound the problem, as we age, we become more sensitive to the effects of these chemicals. That's not surprising. We already have genetic dispositions toward particular diseases and other opportunities to contract all types of diseases, without our own homes adding to the problem!

So, what can you do? You don't need bugs in your life or in your home, but we'll make the assumption that you don't want to kill off your family either. The first thing you can do is to cut down on your usage of these harsh chemical pesticides. You're probably using way too much, too often. The unfortunate result of saturating your yard with these insecticides is that 97% of all the insect life on your residential property are beneficial in nature, actually helping your plant life and the soil itself by increasing its biological activity. The chemicals don't discriminate, however. It's like using napalm.

Pesticides kill off most all life, suffocating and dampening most of the biological activity needed to have a diverse and healthy landscape, with the hopes of ridding you of a small minority of pests. If the products were really good, they would get rid of door-to-door salesmen and nosey neighbors! Instead, you have a bug free, but dead, yard. If you must, limit your use of these products and restrict your pets and children from the yard until the chemical has been watered in properly. Explore some organic products and practices that encourage the use of beneficial insects that may help you in your fight against the minority of unwanted lawn guests. Most large municipalities have been complaining for years about the overuse of these chemicals (it's trickling down into their water supplies), so there is a benefit to the rest of your community for *all* citizens to cut down on the use of commercial insecticides.

Next, if your carpet is old, replacing it may be much simpler than cleaning it properly. If replacing it is not an option, begin by steam cleaning all of your flooring thoroughly. Then, with a hyper-allergenic filter, vacuum the carpeting several times. Going over the same path up to sixteen times has been shown to be enough, according to the same study, to rid the flooring of pesticide residue brought in from the outdoors. I'm sure that seems excessive, but it only has to be done once. After that, clean your pet's paws as they come into your house as best you can, and park your shoes at the door. Also, the use of good mats inside and outside all of your exterior doors helps tremendously. That's a good policy by itself, which will prolong the life of your carpeting tenfold and keep it relatively free of dangerous insecticides. Pesticides can do some real damage to your nervous system; so don't take this lightly, especially if you have small children or elderly adults around.

Mighty Mites

While we're on the subject of carpeting, there lurks another enemy of your health nestled comfortably in your home. A living creature too small to see with the naked eye (there goes that naked eye again), **the dust-mite is not a friend of yours, especially if you suffer from allergies or have a reduced immune system.** If you have respiratory problems several times a year, then dust mites may be unwelcome guests in your home. Do you think that your home is exempt? If you don't have carpeting, draperies, stuffed animals, mattresses, bed coverings and clothing, then you have nothing to worry about. Otherwise, there are probably millions of mites taking up residence with you and paying no rent whatsoever.

Having been around for twenty-three million years, the durable dust mite is only a quarter of a millimeter long. It has eight legs, no eyes, no developed respiratory system, a voracious appetite and can live three to four months. Here's a fun fact; they can produce up to twenty droppings a day (we should be so regular), which means that they are capable of approximately 2,000 feces in their short little lifespan. Theses delectable droppings are what triggers your allergic reaction. As you kick up dust, cleaning and through the normal process of living, these particles become airborne. By inhaling, you ingest the feces into your lungs (what a wonderful thought!). There, they manage to lodge themselves between two adjoining lung cells and break down the walls between them, destroying both cells and causing an allergic reaction…isn't that lovely? Keeping this activity to a minimum would seem to be in your best interest, don't you think?

These little varmints like to eat: human skin scales, molds, pollen grains, bacteria, plant material and the dust containing these materials. One of the ways to get rid of them is to limit the availability of the above-mentioned items. Keeping a clean home is paramount in this battle, but there are several other ways to eliminate them. You can encase bedding materials and pillows in vinyl or plastic for a short period of time. Washing materials in cold water will get rid of the majority of them, but hot water will kill all of them. Dry cleaning also works as does steam cleaning your carpeting. Make sure that you use a dust free bag on your vacuum to keep from recirculating the little devils back into your home. One interesting method to use if you have stuffed animals is to put them in the freezer overnight, which will give the teddy bear a cold but will kill all of the mites that may be residing on Yogi's fur. The mites have no built in protection from sunlight, so keep your drapes open and let as much light in as your utility bill can stand. This will fry them and many other microscopic creatures and bacteria taking up space in your home. They also like moisture, so keep your home "high and dry." Fix all plumbing leaks, use a dehumidifier, and take away their ability to live and function. Look them up on the internet. They are lovely creatures...so lovely that you probably won't lie naked on your carpeting ever again, which is probably a good thing anyway!

Moldy Oldies

The "leprosy" of the new millennium goes by the name of Stachybotrys (stack-ee-*bought*-ris). You say you've never heard of him? Well, his outlaw name is Mold... Black Mold and he's probably in your home right now. Do you need to be concerned? Again, if you have a weak immune system or have any young children running around, then yes, you need to be concerned. If you are going to be selling your home anytime soon, then you may also run into problems. In some parts of the country where mold has become a huge liability issue, home insurance can be very difficult to obtain for properties that have had water problems. A couple of water-based insurance claims and you can forget about finding decent insurance, making your home very difficult to sell, to say the least.

Stachybotrys and his relatives in the mold kingdom have been around as long as Mighty Mite, and like the "too little to be seen" bug, Stachy can be a real problem. He can make some people very sick and theoretically has already killed many thousands. If you live in a dark and musty home, have continuous respiratory problems, suffer from sinuses, colds, flu and other like ailments, then there is a good chance that you are being affected by mold. It mainly affects the very young, the very old and "immunity challenged" people. It may not affect you much at all, but could do some real damage to the ones you love. Chances are, it is at a minimum, compromising your immune system.

What is it? They are simple fungi. They aren't plants, nor are they animals, but they are found all over this planet. (I assume that nature has some productive use for both mold and dust mites, but I'm sure that it has nothing positive to do with mankind.) Of the 100,000 identified fungi, only about 150 are considered toxic . . .

gee, only 150 of them. That's a piece of cake! The problem lies, not so much in the mold itself, but in the spores (seeds) that the mold releases into the air. Then, of course, we breathe the spores into our lungs and before you know it, they are taking up residence with the dust mite feces. (This is getting better and better all the time!)

Stachybotrys is just one of the molds out there, but seems to be the most common and one of the more harmful. It is black in color and like all other molds, needs two things to grow. One is cellulose (a paper or wood product) like sheetrock, and the second is moisture. Your home has plenty of food (cellulous) for the mold; the trick is to keep the other element, the catalyst (moisture) from occurring. Any inside drip, roof leak, and pipe leak inside a wall, any previous water problem not entirely taken care of, any of these can give the mold a chance to grow. If you see a dark stain, you probably already have some mold. If it can be contained, before it spreads the spores, it can be corrected easily. If not, remediation can be very, very expensive. Not only do the remediators have to rip out any of the walls that have the mold, any furniture, clothing, carpeting and other "material" type of things have to be examined and any mold has to be removed from those items. After your entire home has been remediated, all of the "air" inside of your house may have to be exchanged for fresh. That means huge blowers force the air out of your home and then re-circulate new, fresh air back in. No, I'm not kidding. This is a very common step in the elimination of the mold. Unless *all* of the spores are removed from your home including the air inside, there is a good chance that they will reappear. Oh, I forgot to mention . . . you can't live in the home for the several months that this takes to repair your residence, your dry cleaners may not even take your clothes for fear of contaminating their other customers' clothing, apartment managers may refuse to rent you (and your contaminated furniture) a temporary apartment and your insurance company won't be happy to see you when it comes to renewing your policy. No, not kidding about this either. This is an epidemic, of sorts, at least in Texas right now. I know of several people that this has happened to. A friend of mine is still in temporary housing and it's been over three months! He does occasionally get to visit his house, though.

The easy fix to keep this from happening is to look for and repair *any* water leak that you find within a couple of days of the beginning of the leak, seal the stain, or cut it out, and then paint over the repaired section. Take a trip into your attic when it is raining and make sure that your roof isn't leaking. Any time you see water, or evidence of water where it isn't supposed to be, find out what the problem is and get it fixed! You can't get rid of the cellulous, but you can keep the water from becoming the catalyst that starts the process. All of these steps would be the pro-active approach to keeping these problems at a minimum. Remember, this started as an issue with your health. These molds may be a liability issue, but even more important they may be affecting your health without you even knowing it.

Before going any further, it's not necessary to get psychotic trying to eliminate every single bug, every mite and 100% of all fungi from your home. First of all, it is an impossible task. Second, it's not imperative. You can make yourself sick, literally, from the stress of trying to manage these problems and that defeats the entire purpose of pointing them out. You don't have to be obsessive about the cleanliness of your home. Get it clean and keep it that way, keep it picked up, maintain a regular cleaning routine and be aware of the potential problems that exist. After that, don't worry about it, or it will make you nuts.

What you *really* need to do is to increase and maintain a strong immune system that is capable of fighting off any threat that comes your way. With a supercharged immune system, the above-mentioned problems will have a difficult time causing you any distress. By having a "killer" immune system (pardon the pun), you stand the best chance of eliminating most bugs before they have time to get a foothold in your system. The same strong immune system that has been mentioned in the previous chapters that helps prevent disease, slows the aging process, allows your brain to repair and regenerate itself, repairs your vascular system and generally keeps you healthy will also go to bat when it comes to mold, mites and poisons.

Hold the poison, please

And, speaking of poisons, take a look under your sinks . . . the kitchen sink, utility, all of them. Pay careful attention to the multitude of toxic cleaning products that you have bought at different times for particular needs that you probably aren't even using and probably never will. Forget about the danger of your kids or grandkids getting a hold of this stuff. You already know about those types of problems and if you have young rug-rats running around, you probably have the cabinet doors protected from their entry. However, the products themselves don't even need to leave the shelves to do damage to your internal biological system. The products that you have in your home (such as bleach, ammonia products, aerosol cans, insecticides, floor cleaners, toilet bowl cleaners, 409, 509, WD-40, 60, or 80 and all of the rest) can pose potential health risk. By ingesting some of these, either through your lungs, skin or even your digestive system you run the risk of destroying healthy cells, compromising your immune system, and ultimately letting deadly diseases introduce themselves to you. Pesticides, in particular, are now being associated with all sorts of nervous system disorders such as Parkinson's, Alzheimer's, Lou Gehrig's Disease and any other malady having to do with your brain. Chlorine bleach is also bad news. Many of these can release toxic vapors into the air if there is any opening in the container at all (i.e. leaving the container lid cracked or not tight enough, not closing the lid properly, a hairline crack in the bottle's exterior or an old container.) Whatever the case, fumes that you don't need to be breathing could very well be making their way into your lungs. There are so many different chemicals with too many problems to even begin to discuss here. The important thing to realize is that you can get by with a lot fewer cleaning products and their associated chemical ingredients and not sacrifice the cleanliness of your home.

For instance, you can make a "soft scrub" type of cleanser by combining a quarter-cup of all natural baking soda with enough liquid soap to give it the consistency of thin toothpaste. In fact, baking soda, which is sodium bicarbonate, is completely underutilized as a cleaning agent. You can clean your jewelry, silver, countertops, stainless steel and much, much more. A teaspoon of baking soda in a spray bottle of water will get rid of fungus on your houseplants and your rose bushes. Eliminate odors by using baking soda in diaper pails, garbage cans, carpeting, shoes, dishwashers, refrigerators, disposals, and drains. Boost your laundry cleaner's performance by adding a half-cup of baking soda. You can even clean your fruits and vegetables with it!

White distilled vinegar also has a ton of uses. A weak solution in water can clean your countertops, appliances and dishes. Add a couple of drops of liquid dish detergent, a tablespoon of vinegar and fill the rest of a spray bottle with water and you have a great glass cleaner. Use it to keep your bath and shower spotless. A long time "tile man" told me that he won't put anything but vinegar and water on his tile floors. The discoloration of the grout that we all see is a result of soap *and* dirt accumulation, not just dirt. The vinegar cleans, disinfects, and pulls the buildup out of the grout leaving your tile squeaky clean. Clean out your coffee maker, steam iron, washing machine and dishwasher with a strong solution of vinegar. Combine vinegar and baking soda to clean out your plumbing pipes and drains. Disinfect your garbage pails, trashcans, shower curtains and toilets with this nontoxic semi-natural (the white distilled kind) product. A big plus with using baking soda and white distilled vinegar is that they are both extremely inexpensive to use. No, actually they are "dirt" cheap. Pardon the pun, again.

Use olive oil and lemon juice to dust and polish wood. Leave borax in your commode overnight and then flush in the morning to clean. Essential oil of lavender diluted in water is also a good anti-bacterial cleaner. Rub a paste containing salt and vinegar on clothing stains and let sit for thirty minutes. Keep bugs at bay by spreading a thin line of salt across their pathway — they will not cross it.

Most of the rest of the junk in your cabinets are just that . . . unnecessary and unneeded junk. Use up what you have, if you must, and then switch to environmental and people-friendly products and improve your health along the way. If they're old, just throw them out since they may already have gone bad.

Germs, Germs, Everywhere!

Of course, one of the areas of concern in the war against all of the micro-miniature varmints constantly attacking your health is the plethora of germs surrounding you constantly looking for a weakness in your defense. We obviously can't cover all of them, but let's concentrate on the primary ones where we can make a difference.

You're so cold

One is the common cold. We don't have a cure for it and probably won't for some time, but we can sure take steps to minimize their numbers and severity. If you follow the steps outlined in this program and the precautions mentioned in this section, you may never get a cold again. Of course, there are going to be days when you feel exhausted or just plain "puny," but actual colds and cases of the flu may be few and far between. So, let's talk about the cold and some of the ways we can keep the "crud" out of your life.

One of the quickest way to get a cold is to either breathe in somebody else's cold germs or transfer them from a surface that you have recently touched to your mouth or nose, where they can go to work making themselves unwelcome parasites in your body. (Hopefully your now increasingly strengthened immune system will fight off most of them!) The result is usually one more cold than you wanted this year.

Again, strengthening your immune system is the important first step and has been discussed throughout this entire program. Avoidance is the next. The first thing to do is to keep your distance from someone that is in the first three days of having a cold, which is when that person is the most contagious. Unfortunately, you don't usually have that much notice and avoiding them may be difficult.

There is another, almost foolproof, way to avoid unwanted bugs and that is through washing your hands more frequently. Most of us aren't conscious of the number of times we put ourselves at risk of catching colds and viruses by just touching things during our normal day that are contaminated with germs. How many surfaces have you touched today that may have been previously handled by somebody else's snotty fingers? **Every time *you* touch something *you* leave a calling card, your germs. The same holds true for anybody else.** Therein lies the problem. (Actually, the problem isn't the ***touching*** of those items. It's when you then unconsciously touch your fingers to your nose, mouth and eyes, which you will do several dozen times a day. It's tough controlling those activities.) Once the unwanted guests reach those three ports, it's easy sailing from there. Politicians that shake hundreds of hands a day have solved this potential type of risk by having their aids carry disinfectant wipes that they use several times a day. Although there are many hand sanitizers on the market, this may be impractical for you.

How often do you think you come in contact with somebody else's germs? I'll guess that your estimate is way low. Let's go through a normal hypothetical work-day as an example of your efficiency of attracting germs near enough to your internal system to potentially do some damage. We'll begin after you leave your home and are traveling to work and we'll assume that you are driving your own car. If you paid toll, then you may have handled money, which, as you already know, is extremely "dirty" on the germ scale. If not, then you have parked your car and entered your office building by pushing on a door that several other people have already handled. You then may stop off at the bathroom, push on the door to enter, open a stall door and sit down to do your business. When finished, you rearrange your clothes and flush. Hopefully, you then wash your hands with soap before unfortunately again touching the door to get out of the bathroom. You then open at least one and maybe several doors to get to where you actually work, each time handling something that several other people have who may not share your hygiene concerns. Now, needing that first cup of coffee, you open another door or two, pick up the coffee pot, handle the sugar or cream container and maybe pick up a donut that someone else previously examined but then rejected. Repeat that coffee break at least once more before noon. Now, let's not forget about going out to lunch. Open the restaurant door, pull out a chair, pick up a menu, go through the salad bar handling all the utensils needed to make your salad, etc. Venture into their restroom and repeat the same steps you took at your place of employment. Sign your credit card bill with the waiter's pen (carry your own writing utensil is essential), shake hands with the people you dined with and then grab a candy out of the bowl by the hostess stand (which is about the worst violation of the day, given the number of people who have already stuck their hands in that bowl), and then push the door back open to leave.

We have only gotten midway through a typical day and already there have been dozens of opportunities for you to pick up someone else's germs. We haven't even discussed the stapler you used, the telephone, the pen you borrowed, the fax machine, the copier . . . or the boss's face you slapped for the rude comment. Without laboring through the rest of this fairly normal workday, hopefully you can see the potential problems that exist here. **No wonder you get so many colds during the year. Your immune system is constantly working overtime trying to fend off hundreds of attempts to compromise your health daily. Giving your disease fighters a break is very easy to do . . . wash your hands with soap and water several times a day (ten to twelve times a day would be about right). Do that and you will greatly decrease the likelihood of contracting a contagious disease.** At the very least, wash your hands every time you visit the bathroom. I know that seems automatic to most of you, but believe me it's not to everyone, especially men. As we get older we tend to go to the bathroom more often anyway; why not take advantage of opportunity and wash up thoroughly while you're there? Then wash up before and after meals of any kind. You don't even have to use antibacterial soap. Just plain soap and water will do fine. The worst that can happen from this frequent and necessary activity is that you may get dry hands. Big deal. Carry some hand lotion with you if you must. Just don't share it! Does this seem like paranoia and overkill to you? I hope not. **Any doctor worth his or her salt will agree with this assessment and will tell you to wash your hands as many times a day as you possibly can. In fact, the Center for Disease Control and Prevention has called hand washing the "most important means of preventing the spread of infection."** That should be a sufficient enough endorsement. If not, read *any* article written about preventing colds and you will find the same recommendation as being a constant in all of the studies or opinions given.

While we're on the subject of colds, let's offer ten good, general steps to follow that are useful in preventing colds in specific. Although these are excellent overall strategies, they work particularly well in the area of cold prevention.

Top Ten Steps to Cold Prevention

1. Keep your distance from someone just catching a cold.
2. Wash your hands frequently.
3. Get outside more often regardless of the time of year. (It's not the cold weather that makes you sick. It's the confined environment of wintertime.)
4. Sleep long, well and regular. (Live long and prosper too.)
5. Exercise on a regular basis to build your immunity.
6. Gargle at least twice a day.
7. Clean and disinfect any surfaces you come in contact with, often.
8. Consume lots of raw fresh fruits and vegetables each and every day.
9. Hit the vitamin C, increasing the amount that you take daily till you reach 2,500 milligrams.
10. Take zinc and echinecea supplements at the first sign of a cold to shorten its lifespan.

Do these and you will help your body resist infectious illnesses.

Sponge Bob

If you have kids, you know who "Sponge Bob" is. Were our cartoons this stupid? Then there's "Cat/Dog" . . . even dumber. You keep a clean house, right? Probably have a sponge or two lying around to clean up those messes, especially in the kitchen. They may appear clean, but you're probably spreading germs in the process. Researchers at the University of Arizona tested 500 used dishcloths and sponges from five different cities and found that two-thirds of them contained illness-causing bacteria. A quarter of these sponges were hosting staphylococcus and salmonella. (These cause food poisoning, not very pleasant.) About 76 million Americans get food poisoning annually. Of these, approximately 325,000 require hospitalization and 5,000 die. Don't be a statistic! Use paper towels, wash your sponges and dishcloths in the dishwasher or replace them often. A bleach solution will also disinfect them. Again, you just need to be more conscious of the things you can't see that can put you in harm's way. Question: How does one obtain a grant to test sponges and dishrags by traveling around our beautiful country? How do you carry out the study? Do you arbitrarily knock on strangers' doors and ask to see their dish sponges? Sounds like a great gig!

Napalm

Not all of the miniature bugs in your life are bad for you. There are a few exceptions, one being the bacteria that have set up shop in your intestinal tract. They have a direct and very important role in maintaining your health. In fact, they are there by design. From the time you emerged from your mother's womb where you pick up your first set of beneficial bugs, to all of the things you put in your mouth, your system has been collecting these critters to help in the many processes we call life. Most are destroyed when they come into contact with the hydrochloric and other acids produced by your stomach. The few that make it past, settle in your intestinal system and begin their tireless work. Not only do they finish the digestive process allowing the traffic to keep "flowing" down your bucket, they also assist in the manufacture of several important vitamins and enzymes while actually making some on their own. They also fight off the many invasions of your digestive system. Without these, your health will never be as good as it could be. Not only will the essential nutrients pass out of your system without being properly utilized, the lack of the missing enzymes and vitamins will set you up for all sorts of diseases and maladies that will compromise your health and well being. On top of all of that, your entire digestive system will never run as it should, causing you much unnecessary discomfort. These beneficial bacteria are a crucial part of your immune system, and you need to make sure that you protect them, that is, if you still have any. Just as Napalm kills everything in its path, antibiotics eliminate the vast majority of all bacteria in your body. Good or bad, they cannot tell the difference.

When you take antibiotics you accomplish two things: One, you wipe out most of the bacteria that the antibiotic was targeted for, but the collateral damage to the beneficial bacteria is huge. This process eliminates the majority of the good guys crippling their ability to fight off any assault on your system. The second and even more harmful result of antibiotic overuse is that the few surviving "bad" bacteria are now antibiotic resistant and stronger. They begin to multiply by the millions daily and go unchecked since your defensive players have been crippled. Repeat the antibiotic treatment again and they get even stronger. This is survival of the fittest in its purest form! **Because of the complete overuse of antibiotics, there are several strains of antibiotic-resistant bacteria in the U.S. causing the Center for Disease Control to call it an epidemic!** This has caused many fatalities in our country and can be avoided by the proper use of antibiotics.

Most colds and flues are viral based, so antibiotics do absolutely no good. The only benefit, if any, is psychological. You're wasting time and money, and compromising your health by misusing antibiotics. Get off and stay off of them.

"GERMAFRIGERATOR"

Of course that's a word. I just made it up! When's the last time you checked the holding temperature of your refrigerator? We all have leftovers and take-out doggie bags. The question is, "Do we now have more than what we started with? Have our leftovers multiplied?" Many, many workdays missed, many cases of stomach flu and just feeling lousy for a few days are actually cases of food poisoning according to several studies conducted. Whether it's from your favorite restaurant or your favorite refrigerator, it's never pleasant. Check your refrigerator's temperature with a fridge thermometer that you can get at any hardware and some grocery stores. You need to keep it lower than 40 degrees Fahrenheit. Any higher and you're conducting biological experiments.

How long can you keep leftovers in the fridge before they start growing a beard? Use the following guidelines to know when to hold em and know when to fold 'em:

Cooked meats, fish and poultry	3 to 4 days
Raw meats, fish and poultry	1 to 2 days
Luncheon meats (opened)	3 to 5 days
Luncheon meats (unopened)	2 weeks
Eggs (uncooked)	3 weeks
Eggs (cooked)	5 days
Other cooked dishes	3 to 4 days
Anything from your mother-in-law	discard immediately

Home Potpourri

Some general tips before we leave your home, which is beautiful, by the way. Your elegant tastes really show throughout, especially the velvet Elvis above your fireplace!

Protect your hearing. "Huh?" Having trouble hearing, now-a-days? Too many loud concerts when you were younger. I feel your pain, but let's not make it worse. Sounds over 65 decibels can cause general long-term hearing loss. Some household culprits: a blender (90 decibels), hair dryer (95), lawn mower (the same), leaf blower (110), garbage disposal (95) and vacuum (85). I know what you're thinking, and, yes, you still have to run the vacuum. Obviously these modern-day devices are necessary, especially the hair dryer and since they are good exercise, especially the hair dryer, get some earplugs. If you cherish the thought of not being able to hear your spouse . . . just keep on doing what you're doing and tell her the lawn really needs to be mowed every three days!

Be careful mixing drugs and some supplements. Hopefully you won't be on too many prescriptions after following this program, but regarding the few that you may still need to use: make sure, first of all, that all the doctors that are prescribing your meds know all meds you are on along with the supplements that you are taking. Some prescriptions may cancel each other out, some may double the potency of others, and other combinations may be just plain dangerous. Communicate with all your doctors! (By the way, grapefruit juice can speed up the effects of some meds, so don't drink any immediately after taking pills. Don't use St. John's Wort or aspirin before any surgical procedure for entirely different reasons. Although most of the medical community wants to pass judgment on herbs as being relatively worthless, they still want to know all that you are taking. If they are of no supposed value, then why do they care?)

Wear high heels? I think I'm talking to the women, but if not, the same laws apply. That would be the laws of gravity. The laws of gravity state, and I quote, "High heels can hurt you, so don't be stupid, especially if you're overweight." (I've misplaced the physics book that I found that law in, but I'm sure it will turn up somewhere.) High heels do two things. One, they shove a bunch of weight into a point closest to the floor, (that would be your toes) slowly mangling the bones of your feet and ankle, eventually causing immense pain. The only way to repair them is with a surgery that involves cutting the bottom of your foot from heel to toe, and then breaking and reshaping the bones that you have managed to mangle over the last several decades. This surgery also causes immense pain. Several women I know that have had this wonderful surgery would rather give birth a hundred times over again before having this procedure done again! Note: they also had to stay off their feet for six weeks. Second, since your body wasn't designed for this kind of activity, arthritis of the knees is common, which also causes immense pain. If you must, keep the size of the heel under two inches and wear them as little as possible.

Be wary of high-smog alert days. If you live in a big city, near industrial areas, or near polluting factories, etc., stay indoors, (if you can) during these alerts and keep your windows closed. Be careful. As you age, you become more susceptible to the effects of smog and pollution. The pollutants caused by these circumstances put a lot of unnecessary stress on your heart and lungs and this danger is backed up by several studies showing the unhealthy results of this type of an environment. **Exposure can sometimes be as detrimental to your health as puffing on a cigarette for the same amount of time that you are outside.**

Everyone loves to BBQ. However, you now know that most of the foods that normally go on the grill aren't necessarily good for you to consume on a regular basis. You can take some additional steps to lessen the risk of the carcinogens and harmful bacteria caused by the act of heating the meat on a barbecue grill.

Start with scraping and cleaning the grilling surfaces before and after every use. The "gunk" build-up is where the carcinogens are residing. You can still have excellent results with a clean, but maybe not considered "seasoned," grill.

Ground meat, as you know, is a source of harmful bacteria that can make you really ill. The risk can be lessened by adding garlic and onion powder (or flakes) before cooking. The allicin in those two wonderful foods kills most of the bacteria that it comes into contact with. Adding these also has the benefit of improving the taste of the burgers, so use these liberally. (Cherries have the same result.)

Marinate other meats and poultry before cooking them and the risk of carcinogens is greatly reduced. Besides also improving the taste, this process will neutralize bacteria and will break down the fibers of the meat making it easier to chew and digest.

Electromagnetic Fields. Magnetic fields caused by the use of anything electrical (electromagnetic . . . duh!) and by the earth itself pass easily through just about anything, including buildings, manmade structures and human beings like you! In other words, you are being bombarded by tons of these, plus radio waves, twenty-four hours a day! Your microwave, space heaters, television and other appliances generate EMFs. Without going into a lot of detail, the easiest precaution you can take is to stay at least a few feet away from them when in use. Don't stand in front of the microwave while you're waiting for your water to heat. Don't allow your kids to sit two-feet away from the TV. The majority of the magnetic field drops off considerably the farther you get away from the appliance and there should then be no concern for any health issues as long as you stay a reasonable distance away from them.

There is a lot of controversy concerning EMFs. Many studies have shown no ill effects from them. (Most of the studies involve the overhead power lines that so beautifully landscape our cities and towns. Don't buy a house backing to, or next to them. They are hard to resell.) Unfortunately, most of the studies have been sponsored at least in part by the utility companies that have the most to lose if a problem exists. For that reason it would be wise to take those studies with a grain of salt . . . or sugar if you like.

The biggest supposed concern surrounding EMFs has to do with cancer. Many people believe that EMFs, especially the kind generated by power lines, cause all sorts of cancers, especially childhood leukemia and brain cancer. The evidence is weak, but the recommendation would be to avoid them whenever possible just to be sure. Just because no relationship has been found between EMFs and cancer yet, doesn't mean that none exists. This is another situation where you should use your common sense and take the conservative route to a healthy life. Don't rely on the providers of electricity or the federal government to guide your actions in this area. Take charge yourself and don't wait for the evidence to be found *after* you have developed cancer.

Couch taters. While you're on the couch watching that particular appliance throwing magnetic fields your way, please be aware that the longer you stay there (on the couch) the bigger your risk of contracting a life-threatening disease. Harvard University just completed a ten-year study showing that the more television you watch the greater your risk of contracting diabetes. Of the 40,000 men tested, those who watched the most TV tripled their risk compared to the ones who didn't watch much at all. I doubt that EMFs had much to do with the results. It probably had more to do with (the lifestyle) a lack of regular exercise and a poor diet, which cause obesity and thus the pathway to this horrible disease. (The study also showed that the highest risk group tended to eat more risky foods like red meats, processed snacks and basic junk that added to the unhealthy lifestyle leading to the disease.)

The moral of this story is, of course, to get off your butt, go out and work on your yard, walk around your neighborhood or do anything else constructive in nature that keeps you away from the tube. Just don't camp out directly underneath those power lines that are behind your home!

"Didn't I tell you to brush your teeth, young man!"

It turns out your mother was right, for at least one more reason than you (or her, for that matter) previously knew. There have been a couple of studies that have found a relationship between periodontal disease and heart disease. Some of the same plaque that causes gum disease and other mouth problems also has been found to be the culprit in clogged arteries, which leads to obvious problems in your vascular system like heart attacks and strokes. You can look at this two different ways: One, by taking care of your teeth and gums, you may be stopping the spread of harmful bacteria through the rest of your system, or two, the fact that you *have* periodontal problems could be a warning signal to have your entire circulatory system checked. Researchers are not sure whether one or both set of circumstances are correct, so by brushing, flossing and gargling daily you may do more than just keep you spouse from leaving you. **Just another of many examples demonstrating that your body parts all work together and taking care of your entire system is more important than any one piece of the pie, so to speak.**

An aspirin a day keeps Dr. Korvorkian away

You've been reading for years about aspirin's ability to thin your blood just enough and to keep inflammation down sufficiently to significantly reduce your chances for a heart attack. If you're a chronic pain sufferer, then one baby aspirin daily is not a problem. In fact, your blood may be thin enough to seep right through your skin if you eat enough anti-inflammatory pills on a regular basis (don't try that, I was just kidding). For those of you that don't take any over-the-counter drugs, normally that's a good thing. However, this would be an exception. Check with your doctor to make sure there is nothing to get in the way of this small insurance policy. The possible damage that one small baby aspirin daily could do is greatly outweighed by the advantages it offers to your heart.

Part of how aspirin and other nonsteroidal anti-inflammatory drugs work is by blocking an enzyme known as COX-2. By blocking this enzyme, scientists have recently noticed that a lowered risk of colon cancer is also achieved, so it seems that a small dose of aspirin, ibuprofen or naproxen daily will give you an added bonus. Given the relative cost of these products as compared to prescription medication, this is one precaution you shouldn't pass up.

Go Natural

Your home is filled with synthetic products, many of which give off all sorts of wonderful pollutants like formaldehyde and paint residue. Add some beautiful house plants to the mix, and let them filter and eliminate pollutants *and* the carbon dioxide that you exhale while, in return, giving off pure oxygen for you to breathe. All they require from you is a little water and some sunlight. Not a bad deal! Two to three plants per 100 square feet is enough to keep your eyes from itching and help relieve you from asthma and some headaches. The best ones seem to be Boston ferns and ivy, palms and rubber plants. Note: silk plants don't count . . .

Sun Gods

Okay. Now that we have told you to get off your butt and kicked you out of your polluted and dust-mite infested home, be careful not to get too much exposure to ultraviolet rays from the sun. If you are fair-skinned, a red head or blonde, have a history of skin cancer in your family or remember having more than three bad sunburns before you turned twenty, you may be at risk for skin cancer...sorry to be the bearer of less than good news. (A friend of mine from college died at the rather young age of forty from melanoma, so this is not something to mess with.)

Skin cancer is the most common of malignancies in the U.S. and affects more than a million Americans a year. Basal-cell and squamous-cell are the most common and usually affect the face. They can do some real damage to the surrounding tissue and bone, if not taken care of. Melanoma, which is the rarest but most deadly of all skin cancers, has increased tremendously in the last fifty years, probably because of our obsession with the sun (or tanning booths for some.) If melanoma is not caught early, it will spread and greatly reduce your chances to see your grandkid's graduation.

How do you protect yourself? Certainly, if you are in a high-risk category for skin cancer, have your doctor examine you annually and teach you how to examine yourself monthly. (I'm afraid to look at myself...It scares me.) Look for any uneven moles, probably different shades of color that are expanding over time. They will start out being about a quarter of an inch in diameter. (If they get to be as large around as an average umbrella, you should probably make an appointment.)

As far as prevention goes, you probably know the biggies like wearing sunscreen, protective clothing and avoiding the hotter parts of the day. Some other important things to know are as follows: Sunscreen is only good for one season so discard or make pina coladas out of the old and buy some fresh. You need at least SPF 15 or higher if you fit the high-risk category. Although you need about a hour minimum of sun daily, you can get all you need in the morning or after dinner. Leave the rest to the professionals. Wear a broad-rimmed hat and loose fitting, dry clothes. Wet and tight clothes tend to stretch out the fabric, letting in the UV rays. Sunglasses with UV protection are a must any time you're in the sun. Your eyes are very sensitive and can be damaged severely. Here's a new one: Eating a diet rich in beta-carotene like sweet potatoes and carrots can make you twice as resistant to the harmful UV rays of the sun. The pigments that give those foods their rich color can actually build up in your system over time and will give you the protection noted. They are nature's sunscreen. I can't think of a better way to get prepared for tan-time than eating a big bowl of sweet potatoes! (Go light on the toppings, though.) You will still need sunscreen on top of your carrot/potato layer; so don't get too cocky with Mr. Sun. He is the biological father of Mother Nature!

POLLEN AND OTHER WONDERFUL IRRITANTS! OR, "NOT NOW, I HAVE A HEADACHE."

More than forty-five million Americans suffer from chronic headaches and almost 40% of us suffer from some sort of allergies or allergic symptoms, many times causing headaches too. As a result, our economy loses 160 million workdays a year while we spend over two billion dollars annually on over-the-counter pain-killers in an attempt to treat our discomfort. Unfortunately chronic use of over-the-counter pain-killers can cause many other problems including your system becoming resistant to their effectiveness. Many times headache suffers are more disabled than people having chronic arthritis or back pain. When you have a bad headache you're pretty useless to anyone or anything until it shows mercy on you . . . usually by the next morning. Fortunately for you, by following this program the headaches should subside.

An allergic reaction occurs when your immune system mistakes something that is harmless for something that is harmful, the substance causing the adverse reaction being called the allergen. The collateral damage of this particular war is apparent in symptoms you see and feel in your body's bones and soft tissues. These allergens enter your body by inhalation, injection (drug or venom) or swallowing as in foods or drugs. A headache is only one of the symptoms that can arise from allergens.

Allergic reactions often cause headaches, and since the amount of research on the two subjects is overwhelming and beyond the scope of this book, we are going to group them together with migraines. They share many of the same causes. There are two areas we will cover: the avoidance of allergens that are triggering reactions, and building up your immune system to fight off their invasions. (Obviously, headaches caused by a blow to the head, severe muscle strain or extreme stress or tension should be excluded from consideration for the following remedies.)

Nasal congestion (which many times causes the headaches) occurs from one of two reasons. You either have allergic rhinitis, which is an inflammation of the nasal passages due to an allergic reaction, or nonallergic rhinitis being the same inflammation from a nonallergic source. Pretty simple.

Allergic reactions occur from exposure to: animal dander, house dust, fungal spores, grasses, specific types of foods, dust mites, pollens and feather pillows to name a few. Ridding yourself of the above-mentioned triggers might reduce any symptoms that you have. If you have eliminated most and still suffer from allergies of some sort, then it may be time to have some sophisticated food allergy tests done to rule out specific foods as the culprits. Many food allergens include: package foods containing processed fats and nitrates, caffeine, chocolates, certain nuts, dairy products, shellfish, and soy. Don't eliminate these from your diet until you have been tested, though, since many of these are good for you. (Many children on Ritalin for A.D.D. are found later to suffer from food allergies only . . . and are then removed from the drug.)

You can have nonallergic reactions to many things in your personal environment. These include: temperature change, air pollutants of all sorts, gasoline, paint or chemical fumes, perfumes, alcohol-especially red wines, cigarette smoke and in-laws. Take steps to eliminate or avoid these and your life may become more bearable. For instance, when your mother-in-law comes over, go golfing or to the nearest watering hole until she leaves! Many of these irritants are probably obvious to you and you may know within seconds if something in particular is giving you a headache.

On the other hand, many allergens are less obvious. Studies have shown that the inside of your home is a lot more polluted than outside. One of the main reasons is that newer homes are so airtight that normal out-gassing that should occur doesn't because the gasses have nowhere to go. They are wrapped and insulated probably too well, not allowing the proper re-circulation of air. Your dishwasher, washing machine and showerheads, for instance, do a great job vaporizing some harmful chlorination by-products into the air, which you then inhale. Your exposure to toxic chemicals is then greater from taking a shower than from drinking a glass of tap water. If you're concerned about the water that you drink, then you should also be aware of the potential problems with the water particles that you inhale. The fix here is to put carbon filters on your showerheads and ventilate by opening windows or turning on exhaust fans when operating the other appliances. You may not have an allergic reaction to these substances, but they could contribute to the weakening of your immune system. Similarly, candles, especially scented ones should not be burned. Not only are the soot particles just small enough to be deposited in your lungs and the accompanying carcinogens may travel into your bloodstream, they also do a very good job of ruining the paint on your walls and ceilings. Use potpourri instead.

Headaches and allergies are not only a nuisance or a discomfort, there is new evidence that they can interfere with your immune system allowing diseases of many types to gain a foothold in your system so you want to take steps to eliminate these as much as is possible.

Take the following ten steps to rid yourself of the majority of triggers that may cause discomfort in the form of an allergic reaction and/or a headache. Some of these are general in nature, but are extremely important in your fight against allergies and headaches.

Ten Steps to Allergy Relief

1. Use HEPA (high-efficiency particulate) filters on your air conditioning system and vacuum cleaner.
2. Keep your home light, bright and clean including vacuuming at least weekly.
3. Replace old carpeting and draperies and use tile and hardwoods whenever possible to limit carpeting in your home.
4. Improve your diet, concentrating on fresh fruits and vegetables. Include apples, onions, garlic, apple cider vinegar, local raised honey and alfalfa or "green food" supplements. Exclude dairy, red meat, processed foods and caffeine as much as possible.
5. Begin and stay on an exercise program concentrating on cardiovascular (aerobic) routines.
6. Wash bed linens and towels in hot water weekly.
7. Pollen is usually released in the morning, so stay inside if necessary.
8. Keep your pets out of your bedroom.
9. Get tested for food allergies, if necessary. Let your doctor know all of the medicines and supplements that you are taking.
10. A good night's sleep is imperative. Get at least eight hours.

The main thing that you can do is to increase your awareness of the your immediate surroundings, your personal environment, and follow the practice of avoidance whenever possible. Hopefully, what you have just read will help. Also remember that all of the over-the-counter products that you take to dull the pain, do just that. They do not cure or get rid of the problem. They are merely a temporary solution, nothing more than a band-aid.

A long and slow death

Smoking and drinking have been mentioned several times for obvious reasons. Live a life chock-full of smokes and booze and you will not live as long or as comfortably, pure and simple. Since this section is about the "defensive driving" of your life, mentioning these two again is only natural.

Drinking eats out and renders your liver useless. Upward of 35% of all drinkers have some sort of alcohol-related liver problems. Unfortunately God insisted that you have and use one. And God said, "On the sixth and one-half day, I threw in some liver (and onions) to balance man's body so he wouldn't list to one side." Just so you would know it was there, he made it the biggest of all your organs (not including your skin) and made sure that everything that entered into your body was filtered through your liver. No liver, no filtering, no enzyme production, no good health, etc . . . You need your liver so cut down or quit (if you have a drinking problem) entirely. It will kill you prematurely.

Smokers are twenty-five times more likely to die from lung cancer as non-smokers. (Not a stretch of imagination here!) They are three times more likely to die of a heart attack than a healthy person, and besides their scratchy voices, their clothes stink too. Their skin will be thinner and less elastic, they will turn gray four-times sooner, so while they are dieing sooner, they will also look the part. Let's not forget the wrinkles around their mouths they got from sucking on cigarettes for the last thirty years. Lovely.

Bottom line is that this entire chapter (and this complete program for that matter) is a waste of time to the smoker and/or drinker who aren't planning on quitting. All the preventative care in the world cannot overcome the ill effects of smoke and alcohol. It will destroy your marriage, your career, any good relationships you have developed and ultimately your life. But you'll have a fun time doing it!

Nympho-Lympho

Have you given your lymphatic system a hug recently? Have you told it how much you appreciate the hard work it's doing? Probably not. In fact, you more than likely don't *ever* think of it, nor even know what the heck it does. The only time you hear about it is in a bad context as in, "Well, John has got stomach cancer and it has reached his lymph nodes." From that statement you know that John's time on this planet is short because cancer hitting the lymph nodes is like sending it at warp-speed throughout your system.

The truth is, that if you made it a point to take good care of your lymphatic system, there's a good chance that you would live longer . . . and adding percentage points to the possibility of you extending your life is what this program is all about.

So, just what the heck does this system do? Have you ever been to Disneyland or Disney World? Ever noticed how clean the entire complex is, but you seldom ever see any signs of major cleanup activity other than an occasional maintenance worker sweeping up debris? That's because they have an entire network of underground tunnels that snake through the park carrying most of the workers, maintenance equipment and trash. They are hard at work twenty-four hours a day, but you never see them.

Your lymphatic system is just that. It's the BFI (a very large trash collection company) of your body, among other responsibilities. You actually have *two* circulatory systems. One is the blood carrying, heart pumping system you know all about, the lymphatic system is the one you seldom hear of, even though its larger in fluid than the blood system and equally as crucial. This most important system of your immune function is a network of vessels and nodes filled with fluid that sweeps toxins from in and around your cells, removes infectious organisms and sends these and any other harmful substances on their merry way to your liver and kidneys for processing, before *those* organs sweep the unwanted aliens to that porcelain god outside of your body. (Or if you're a guy, then behind that Buick at the far end of the parking lot.)

Imagine, if you will, your system of arteries and veins snaking throughout your entire body and you've got a good picture of where your lymphatic system is located. It's everywhere your blood is. There are also hundreds of nodes situated at key point along the system, most in your neck and chest area, that are loaded with cells that attack, trap and kill invading germs as they go by and them send them on for punishment. The nodes are also like transfer stations, holding tanks for many of your immune fighters and a temporary jail for the offenders.

Another function of this system is to assist in the nourishment of your body. Blood and sugar (glucose) that have traveled through your arteries and into smaller capillaries are then forced out of the vessels, through lymph fluids and swept into each and every one of your cells for nourishment, energy production and waste control (mine comes every Tuesday morning usually before lunch, but the recyclables only twice a month). The metabolites and lactic acid, among the waste particles accumulated, pass back through the lymphatic fluid and back into the blood system for cleansing.

The problem with this system is that the collection of waste is not perfect (for those of you that thought you were perfect, here's proof that you are not) and a fairly large residue of harmful substances is left in the lymph canals. If your lymphatic system is sufficiently strong, then the unwanted poisons will make their way through the system and to the central processing plant (where all the garbage trucks end up at the end of the day), yours being located in your chest and called the thoracic duct. Here, the remaining waste is dumped back into your bloodstream and ends up taking a short trip to be processed by your liver and kidneys . . . kind of a double-check system.

Why are we discussing your lymphatic system in the Defensive Driving section of this program? Besides having nowhere else to put it, you actually *do* have some control over its efficiency, so consider the taking care of your lymph network as good preventative maintenance. This system is all too important in maintaining your immune system, among other things to ignore. It's like the exhaust system on your car. You never consider it at all, but try stuffing some rags up your exhaust pipe (your car's exhaust pipe!) and see how long your vehicle will run. Not very, because it will get so stopped up that the motor will choke to death. Disconnect the exhaust system entirely and your entire neighborhood will know when you arrive home by the noise . . . along with a glove box full of traffic tickets to boot.

If you are following the principles of this program, then hopefully you are taking fairly good care of your lymphatic system now, but there is still more that you can do. Oh boy! More stuff to do! Aren't you excited? It's not real difficult stuff. Most of the fortifying is easy to do. All you really need to do is to hang upside down, like a bat, using an inversion system for about twenty minutes a day and that should reverse the flow of the stopped up lymphatic sewer gunk stopping up your body. (Make sure to bounce up and down several times.) Then when you stand back up straight, the light headed sensation you have is just the rush of waste cascading toward your liver and kidneys . . . so you might want to stay close to a bathroom. Just kidding, again. Actually, hanging upside down is good for you, and if you ***do*** have a chin-up bar and the boots needed, go for it! Otherwise, there are some more practical activities to partake in that will do just fine. Like, can you take deep breaths? Deep breathing will actually "need" and massage the fluids along the system. Remember that most of the nodes and the thoracic duct are in your chest region; so the deep breathing that you need to do anyway will help this system. While you're walking or doing certain exercises, take those deep breaths. How about while you're reading? Anytime that you think of it, breath deeply. It's good for you. You only need about ten minutes of deep breathing a day to make a difference. Your lymphatic system has no heart, or pumping system of any kind, so it needs other pressures to move the fluids along. Aerobic type of exercising is particularly beneficial. Those mini-trampolines are great. Basketball, jumping rope, calisthenics, wild sex (doing, not watching), martial arts, or anything that bounces you around will move the lymphatic fluids where they need to go.

You need an excuse to give and get massages, don't you? Well, a good rubdown, especially a neck and upper body massage will do wonders for this bodily function besides all the other physical and emotional benefits of this activity. The actual deep massaging will physically move the fluids along the vessels and keep them clean. Go rub somebody . . . hopefully not the wrong way.

Stand up straight, young man. Ah yes, I still remember those words. Unfortunately, they were words of wisdom not heeded as a child. Now, as a big child, those words have a lot more meaning. Hunching over does the lymphatic system no good. Having correct posture will allow the system to have a better chance to function properly. That's common sense, if you stop and think about it. Allowing your body to stretch out straight will open up the canals so that they can move the fluids along. It's like having your leg "fall asleep" on you when you position your legs in such a manner to cut off the flow of blood. Stand tall, take deep breaths and save your spinal structure while you're at it.

Also having a good diet and getting regular plus sufficient sleep is extremely helpful. Those are steps that you should already be taking for other reasons previously discussed. Now you have one more *very* good excuse. Again, all functions of your body are related in some way, and this is no exception.

Can it!

The aluminum can revolutionized the soft drink and beer industries. Unfortunately it's time to make some changes. The aluminum in the cans (also in aluminum cookware) can leach into the drink inside and then, of course, into your system. No problem except aluminum in excess is toxic. Research has shown that excess aluminum causes brain cells (they used the proverbial rat for the study . . . they couldn't find any humans dumb enough to let them inject aluminum into their blood system.) to lose their ability to absorb glucose, which is their energy source. Without glucose, dementia settles in, a symptom of Alzheimer's, Lou Gehrig's disease and Parkinson's disease. See any relationships here?

There are so many *little* things that can contribute to symptoms normally associated with aging, especially neurological problems. This is an example of one of the "little things" that you can do to stave off Father Time. No one is going to stop using all aluminum cans, but it's easy enough to substitute plastic bottles or fountain drinks when available. You can switch at home, most convenience stores sell both and they are generally less expensive than aluminum cans. Improve the taste of the beer that you drink by switching to bottles, too.

Again, at home, don't let aluminum foil come in contact with whatever it is that you are storing, don't use aluminum pots and pans and keep acidic foods clear of this product. (Acidic foods leach the aluminum more efficiently.)

While you're at it, stay away from certain antacids, baking powder, some teas, and any processed foods that contain aluminum. Oh, your tap water probably contains a trace amount too. Switch to distilled or highly-filtered H_2O when you can.

The study of the effects of aluminum on your body is fairly new with not a lot of hard data available at the present, but why take any chances. Keeping excess toxins away from your body is just some more common sense. Again, we don't want to wait for the incriminating evidence to show up after using an abundance of aluminum cans for the last forty years.

"I'M IN A NEW YORK STATE OF MIND"

As it was sung by Billy Joel. He was born a New Yorker and will probably call it home for the rest of his life. Maybe you feel the same about the area that you reside in. Your friends live there and/or your family could be entrenched there. It could be that you love the weather. All of those things are important and may be vital to your overall emotional health and physical well-being. You may, however, want to consider *all* of the aspects of where you live. Not just the amount of friends that also call this their home, but all of the other physical aspects of your region like pollution of all types, the kind of industries that are concentrated there, the amount of traffic congestion, the cultural opportunities, the rate of crime, etc. The results of all of these thrown in with other factors are assimilated by companies that care . . . like the insurance industry. They care because they want to know when you are going to die, even more so than Lenny, your conniving nephew that thinks he is getting a piece of your pie.

What's important here is whether or not living where you do is healthy for you. Yes, it does matter and the statistics consistently show that **where you live is maybe as important as how you live.** Insurance statistics taken on the following conditions demonstrate some interesting results. The number of deaths in each state from cancer, infant mortality, diabetes-related ***and*** overall deaths per

100,000 residents is fairly consistent from state to state. States that had high rates of death in one area had elevated numbers in other indicators also.

The winners, according to the many factors used? Not surprisingly, the best state to live in is Hawaii. Warm weather, lots of sunshine, an abundance of fish, fresh fruits and vegetables and a really, really low level of stress all contribute to their longevity. Okay, maybe Hawaii is not based in reality. The best flags to live under stateside are Utah, California and Colorado. It could very well have something to do with the average resident's lifestyle and the amount of time spent outdoors. You'll notice that two of the three are in cold climates and California has some of the worst pollution in the country, but the other factors outweigh some of the negative ones. When I think of these three states, I think of people more concerned with their health than in the rest of our country. They bike, ski, hike and spend time outdoors, all of which are important factors in overall health.

Which, do you think, are the most dangerous states to live in? One of the first ones kind of surprised me. The District of Columbia and Louisiana are both at the top (or bottom, if you prefer) of this list. D.C. probably because of the high crime rate, the obvious stress caused by being at the heart of our nation's capital *and* being around so many lawyers . . . all with mile-long egos! It's enough to drive you to drink, which is probably what happens.

I assumed Louisiana to be the most deadly state in our union and the research proved me correct. The Bayou state, unfortunately, is the cancer capital of the United States. A portion of the reason is that half of our entire nation dumps their pesticide residue, chemical poisons, human waste and other undesirables into the Mississippi River and guess where it ends its journey? New Orleans . . . or at least, close by. Add in the poverty, the party atmosphere of New Orleans and the surrounding area, hurricanes and tornadoes, and all of the fattening Cajun food and you have a recipe for failure. They cannot even bury their dead underground in New Orleans! The above-ground burial vaults are a strange site. Louisiana is a great place to go and have a great time. Just make sure you go back to Pueblo when you're done.

Where you live is very important to your health and at least having the information available is paramount. You can find out how your state faired by going to www.statehealthfacts.kff.org. I sincerely hope that you aren't living on top of a radioactive dumping site, near Three Mile Island, next to oil refineries or in a mobile home park smack dab in the middle of tornado alley! It may be time to buy that second home.

Where you live, how you live, what you surround yourself with and how well you take care of your personal environment are just a few of the factors that can contribute to your overall health and well being. By taking precautions and being aware of your surroundings, you can do a lot to affect the time you have left on this planet. Take a real close look at your home, keep the pesticides and other poisons away, insulate yourself from microorganisms that want to do you harm and remember to drive with your eyes wide open.

Step 8:

Water, Life's Elixir

Approximately 75% of our earth is covered with water *and* 75% of your body is made up of water. Coincidence? Probably not. You are *"of this earth"* as you have heard from other sources, which rings true when discussing the relationship of your body's need for clean fresh water.

Plain old boring water is the *most abundant* and *most important* substance in your body. You can "live" without vitamin C for a long time. The same for potassium and all the other vitamins and minerals, but deprive your body of all sources of water and you will perish rather quickly. You can survive several weeks without food, but only a few days without water.

In fact, without it, all the nutrients in the world will do absolutely no good, even if you try and ingest them dry . . . with no water.

Water regulates every function in your body. It carries *all* of the valuable nutrients discussed above to each and every cell in your system. It transports oxygen *to* your cells and toxins *away* through your blood and lymphatic systems, both of which are

mainly H_2O. It's the lubricant that cushions your joints and protects your organs and every tissue from trauma and shock. Your brain is almost 85% water and its not surprising that all neurotransmitters are delivered to nerve endings from your head all the way to your little pinky toes on waterways. Without enough water, your body temperature would spike tremendously, you could not digest your food properly and your muscles would freeze up terribly, among other wonderful effects.

It's safe to say that you do not get enough water. You may consume enough liquids, but many of them like coffee, sodas and alcohol are diuretics and will take water *away* from your system. **Research indicates that most symptoms of aging are a result of dehydration of your organs, tissues, *and* damage done by free radical oxygen molecules roaming around your body. The symptoms of arthritis, allergies, constipation, high blood pressure, back pain, migraines, stress and depression manifest themselves many times from dehydration alone.** A water-retention problem (edema), as an example, is your kidney's attempt to conserve water because of an imbalance of minerals, not a result of drinking too much. Your first reaction would be to stop drinking water to get rid of the bloated feeling. However, the real solution is to drink *more* water, not less, and balance the minerals in your body. When do you need water? How about when your mouth is dry? Sorry, by the time that symptom occurs, it's usually too late. Unfortunately, dry mouth is one of the last indications that you are becoming dehydrated. You have probably lost two cups of water by then. Losing as little as 5% of your bodily fluids can cause headaches, fatigue, confusion and an elevated heartbeat. That's why you need to be continually supplying your system with enough water to keep everything "greased, lubricated" and running smoothly.

Your cells actually become dehydrated as you age. Every cell in your body contains and is also surrounded by water. The ratio of this relationship when you were young was about one to one.

In other words, there was approximately as much water inside of each cell as there was outside. This allowed for the proper exchange of nutrients and waste in and out of each and every cell on a continuous basis through osmosis. As you age and continually reduce your consumption or retention of water that relationship diminishes, and by the time you reach senior citizen status, that ratio can shrink to as low as .8 to 1, which means that there is more water outside of your cells than inside. Your cells become very inefficient and problems arise. You become dehydrated at the cellular level, which manifests itself in disease or symptoms of disease! Instead of treating these problems with water, we visit our doctor and receive prescription medication, which may further mask these symptoms and probably won't get rid of the underlying dehydration problem.

It has been estimated that 75% of us don't drink enough H_2O, (generally speaking, enough is only eight glasses a day). We fill up on coffee, snacks, sodas and tea and don't usually get even enough liquid volume out of these. Are you hungry? Many times hunger pains are only your body's cry for more water. Instead, you go for the Snickers bar and compound the problem in other ways. Drink water at the first sign of hunger and lose excess weight the easy way.

Most older people don't consume enough water. Perhaps they just don't think about it or maybe they're afraid of having frequent urination problems. They may have a loss of thirst and appetite, but whatever the reason, they are compounding their aging process by depriving their systems of the most valuable element they need. The brains of people having died as a result of Alzheimer's have been found to be shriveled up because of dehydration. It makes you wonder how may lives could at least be prolonged by prescribing water instead of drugs that are used to treat symptoms and not the cause. That is not to say that Alzheimer's can be cured by just drinking more water. However, the evidence points toward water's ability to at least relieve symptoms of this and many other ailments.

Water is a solvent. It regulates every function in your body. It carries every element your body needs to operate correctly, and once those things get to where they are supposed to, water controls their activity. All of your organs are nurtured by H_2O; they in turn manufacture hormones, enzymes, acids, vitamins and other beneficial chemicals that are then transported back through your body using . . . you guessed it, water!

The biggest problem with water is that it is virtually free and readily available. There is no special interest group, association or industry to recommend it, promote it, and sell its virtues. Nobody can make a living selling you tap water. Sure, you can buy all sorts of exotic waters, when all you need is good tap water or maybe inexpensive filtered water. For your doctor to just tell you to drink more water would seem to be an insult to your intelligence. You made an appointment, sat in his office for an hour, paid him a lot of money and he tells you to drink water. "Where's the expensive, side-effect causing drug?" you ask. "Nope, don't need it," Dr. Welby says . . . That just ain't gonna happen.

Let this be another instance of you taking control of your health. There really is only one special interest group that will properly and objectively look out for your well-being and that is you. The "Me, Myself, & I Association," starring you as CEO. Start drinking more water today!

DIGESTIVE PROBLEMS

Heartburn, gastritis, constipation, colitis and cancers of this region can many times be avoided by increasing your intake of water alone. The more water that you consume, the more of a certain enzyme called motilin is produced that causes the rhythmic contractions in your intestines. This obviously keeps things moving along. Keep the traffic in your digestive system from becoming a traffic jam by simply drinking more H_2O. Constipation, besides being a royal pain, can also be a major league symptom of severe and potentially life-threatening diseases. Many times it is caused by just a lack of water.

One of the functions of your large intestine is to remove excess water out of . . . out of . . . let's just call it "your waste" . . . and speed "it" on its merry way. When there is dehydration in the rest of your body, there is a demand to pull moisture out of your bodily waste and send it to help, which causes "your waste" to become hard, slowing down its passage to the land of the sewer Gods. The less-than-surprising result is constipation. If this happens too often and for too long, the deposits left on your intestinal walls can cause problems such as diverticulitis and colon cancer. Diverticulitis is bulges or sacs pressing out of your intestinal walls. These sacs will accumulate waste causing all sorts of pain and problems, especially if one bursts. Basically, your waste, with the aid of fiber (which also scrubs and cleanses your intestinal walls) and water, should make its way through your system quickly so that your intestinal walls remain clean and free of any buildup of waste or you're inviting future problems. Water helps alleviate these types of problems.

ARTHRITIS

Millions of Americans suffer from many forms of arthritis. The numbers are staggering. Almost fifty million Americans have arthritis today and the problem is quickly getting worse.

As you probably know, bones that intersect each other are protected by cartilage attached on each side of the bone so that the bones do not rub into one another. This cartilage contains a high level of water, which greatly assist the lubricating process. In fact, you could say that water is the lubricating mechanism! As the cartilage surfaces glide over each other, some of the surface cells die and are hopefully carried away from your system (by water, of course). You also hope that new cells are generated to make up for the ones lost in the normal process of movement in the joint. These prospective cells come from the growing ends attached to your bones. They grow out from the bone towards the joint. It's similar to your finger or toenails. Growth comes from the inside/out. Your exterior nails continuously grow. The only difference is that you can't bite off the cartilage in your joints like you do your fingernails!

There is a built-in problem. It has to do with the "pecking order" or prioritized needs of water in your body. The water needed to nourish the cartilage in your joints comes from the same source that nourishes and encourages the blood cells in your bone marrow. In short, your body determines that your bone marrow takes priority over cartilage production in a dehydration state. No water, no cartilage production and your joints eventually wear out. Pure and simple. Give yourself enough water to nourish both your bone marrow and joint cartilage

Caffeine and diet sodas

As you already know, caffeine is a diuretic, meaning that it causes you to flush water out of your system. Obviously, if you need eight glasses of water a day and instead, substitute caffeinated sodas, you won't be getting enough water. However, there are plenty of other problems associated with an over-use of caffeinated drinks of all types including sodas, tea and coffee.

By the mid nineties, Americans consumed fifty gallons of soda a year, almost 30% of those being of the diet variety. That's a lot of Cokes! Thirty-five gallons of sugar-laced drinks plus a truck-load of caffeine and we wonder why we're in lousy shape? Teeth rotting, gut rotting, brain rotting, carburetor rotting and floorboards rotting. Throw your stock portfolio in and everything is rotting!

Trying to lose weight by drinking tons of diet sodas is a mistake. Overeating is an unfortunate byproduct of drinking diet sodas because of your brain's confusion over thirst and hunger sensations. Your mind thinks it is still hungry instead of only requiring water. The technical reasons have to do with energy conversion in your cells and the chemicals that aspartame (the artificial sweetener in sodas) produce. When aspartame is processed, your brain actually uses more of its energy reserves than necessary, which stimulates hunger signals. So, if you have a sedentary lifestyle and consume a lot of diet sodas, you will probably gain, instead of lose weight. Also, a bi-product of aspartame is its conversion in your digestive tract to methyl alcohol/formaldehyde, or wood alcohol! Lovely, huh! Although drinking a few diet drinks may not kill you, controlling its consumption will benefit you greatly. If you are one of the many people that react harshly to aspartame, then you need to stay off of soft drinks entirely. In fact, your health would probably improve by eliminating aspartame altogether.

Hypertension (High blood pressure)

Water plays a crucial role in regulating the amount of pressure applied to the walls of your blood vessels. Too much pressure and you have the condition known as high blood pressure. Not a big deal, though. All it really can do is give you a stroke, heart attack or just plain kill you. But let's not sweat the little details.

What is water's role? When the total fluid volume in your body decreases, your main blood vessels also have to decrease their aperture (shrink down in size) to compensate for the loss of volume. If too severe, or for too long a period of time, dehydration places an unhealthy amount of pressure on the remaining vessels. This process of re-allocating blood goes on all the time and for the most part is normal. Many of your tiniest blood vessels open and close to help regulate the amount of water available and the pressure exerted within the complete blood system. Imagine opening and closing the smallest tributaries of the Mississippi River to control the level of the big river itself. Your body works in a similar fashion. Another example involves blood being reallocated when you eat. It is redirected to your digestive system in order to help in the process and then sent away after the digestion has been completed. That is why you sometimes feel tired after eating. Some blood has literally left your brain.

Getting a sufficient amount of exercise is also important to mention here. The more your muscles are exhausted through exercise, the more capillaries will open and therefore hold a greater volume of blood within your circulatory system. The greater volume of blood in these vessels will result in less pressure being exerted upon the entire system. The moral here, of course, is to exercise and drink plenty of water.

WATER TYPES

There are several other problems associated with not getting enough water daily, but hopefully now you can see how important hydration is to your system without delving into other boring biology lessons. That brings us to the next question and that has to do with the "type" of water you should drink. I know, I can hear you now. "Not only do I need to drink **more** water, but now I have to drink a specific **type** of water!" If you're highly sensitive to allergens, smoke and basically anything in your personal environment, the type of water you drink **will** make a difference.

In a perfect world you could walk down to any stream, fill your water bottle and drink away. That obviously is not a good choice today. I have a friend living in Aspen, Colorado that has told me the water in the pools at the top of their majestic mountains isn't even good to drink without treating it chemically first. If you can't drink *that* water without treating it first, then there probably aren't any above-ground water sources in America fit enough to be used as they are found naturally. That's a shame, but unfortunately is a reality in our increasingly polluted world.

How good is your local water source? It probably "passes" federal allowances for impurities including: poisons, pesticides, carcinogens, animal and human waste, farm runoff, petroleum products and let's not forget illegal dumping of anything else that has made it to your faucet. Your water treatment plant more than likely does a good job of filtering most of those impurities out, but is it good enough? I'm not so sure I want to trust our government "standards" when it comes to my overall health. A certain "parts per million" of Dursban (a pesticide) may be okay for some of us, but how is your body going to react to it? We all have enough outside, negative factors bombarding our system on a daily basis without having to worry about the water that we drink too.

The purest water that you can get is distilled. Distilling water removes virtually 100 % of all impurities. You can't get better than that. There is no doubt that drinking mostly distilled water will be the very best way to re-hydrate your system, but that may not be practical. Remember, part of this program is based on practicality and finding distilled water all the time would be very difficult. The next best water source for your needs is reverse osmosis and/or highly filtered through a carbon filter. Both share pretty similar results and remove a high percentage of chlorine, fluoride and any other particles. These processes don't remove 100% of the existing impurities, but they get pretty close. They get close enough to perfection and are readily available enough to warrant either as your primary source of water.

Whether it's from a built in refrigerator water dispenser, a table-top filter system, a faucet-connected model, or purchased at a store, if you make an effort, then drinking "better" water **can** and **will** happen. Arguments can be made all day about your liver and kidneys ability to filter regular tap water sufficiently, but we're going to make the assumption that you have abused those two organs sufficiently enough to justify giving them a break whenever you can. This is one of those chances. Pure, clean and fresh water is what your body wants more than anything else and it's up to you to comply. (Note: Don't pass up drinking water entirely when all that is available is from a drinking fountain or some other non-filtered source. The main point is to continually drink water; just attempt to drink distilled or filtered when possible.)

If you use a filtration system, don't forget to change the filters or do the maintenance when needed. Use clean and sanitized glasses, holding containers and make sure anything you come into contact with in the process of getting fresh water is clean. Water's downside is that it will spoil easily if microbes come in contact with it.

Now that you have seen in black and white many of the reasons why, it's time to make water more of a priority in your life. Drinking more pure and fresh water from clean and filtered sources will go a long way in improving the efficiency of all of your internal systems, the processes of manufacturing vitamins, hormones, and enzymes, and will inhibit dementia and other neurological disorders from becoming a part of your life, now or later. Use it as a diet aid, to relieve arthritic discomfort, to regulate blood pressure and to balance and maintain the minerals you desperately need. Your body will thank you.

Step 9:

It's All in Your Mind, Have a Nice Day

At least 80% of this program has to do with the building and fortifying of your immune system. If you have a strong and sound defense system you will probably live to be a ripe old age and relatively free of most diseases and ailments. **You wouldn't think that your brain would have a whole lot to do with the performance of your immune system, but countless research has shown that what goes on in your noggin has as much to do with you staying healthy as any food you eat or exercise you perform.** You are about to find out many of the tools you possess above your shoulders that can extend your life and keep you, and the area south of your neck healthy.

When we talk about you taking control of your health, we're generally referring to you taking some sort of action, whether it is starting an exercise program, having certain precautionary tests run, or guarding the quality of sleep that your body requires.

Equally important though has to do with your attitude about your health, your will and desire to live a long and happy life and your outlook on the world around you. Why? Your life literally depends on it.

The human heart, lungs and liver may be a deck of card's jack, queen and king respectively, but the mind is the ace of spades. As important as all your organs are, they are obviously nothing without your brain. It is your nerve center, it directly or indirectly controls just about everything that goes on in your system, and without it, life ceases to exist for all intents and purposes. Look at someone that has been classified as brain dead . . . no, not your brother-in-law. Maybe someone that has had the oxygen cut off from his brain for longer than a few minutes and has no brain activity left. He may be breathing, but he isn't really living. Once the brain dies, it's all over and you pass to the other side. No mulligan, no get out of jail card and no free pass. End of story.

Besides all of the conscious functions that your brain controls, there are many, many roles it manages that keeps you alive and generally healthy. Hormones and chemicals of all types are manufactured and regulated by your brain that control everything from the amount of pain you are capable of feeling to your success at beating many diseases from arthritis to cancer.

Perhaps the best way to show how your mind can help you beat Father Time is to first look at what it can do to take you down and whittle away at your health. Whether it be from adding an occasional cold or flu to putting an "open for business" sign in front of cancer cells allowing them to gain a strong foothold in your system, your mind is very capable of affecting the rest of your life. **That being said, within reason, you can literally control how long you live and how healthy you will be by the way you live your life.** Mother Theresa and George Burns both lived forever; Scrooge died at the age of 27 and Darth Vader expired when he was 22. Countless studies show that happy people live longer than folks who aren't.

Seen anybody with road rage? Not only are *those* people involved in more traffic fatalities than the more serene drivers, they are also more likely to have psychological and substance abuse problems. Is this an example of the chicken or the egg question? Did the psychological deficiencies cause the *intermittent explosive behavior,* as it is called, or did the behavior manifest itself first? Good question.

Along those similar lines, are you, or do you know, people who are generally angry? The VA studied them several years ago and found out that they were more likely to develop angina or coronary heart disease. In fact, they were two to three times more likely to suffer these even after adjusting out cigarette smoking and other risk factors. This is not difficult to understand. Over time, the cortisol that is constantly released when you are angry damages the lining of your blood vessels and oxygen-rich organs like your heart and eyes.

The American Journal of Preventative Medicine reported that men and women (more often in women) that have been abused either physically or mentally by their partners were more likely to develop health problems later in life than the normal population. These include substance abuse, general mental illnesses and actually sustaining serious physical injuries. Again, this is a no-brainer in understanding that this can occur. The actual chemical changes that happen are probably more complicated, but realizing the relationship is the important point to make.

THE TEAM

This would be a good time to take a tour of your immune system factories and see how your management team meshes them all together. Your immune system is actually a rather complex network of organs (the factories) that manufacture different cells (your foot-soldiers) that do the actual hand-to-hand combat against the things that wish to do you harm, like telemarketers.

Your B-cells consisting mostly of immunoglobulins, (God bless you) are proteins that constantly circulate in your blood supply and other fluids attacking invading bacteria, inhaled pollens and foreign red blood cells. They are your perimeter defense, your body's initial response against antigens. T-cells and various white blood cells communicate with the rest of your immune system while delivering hopefully the final blow to whatever it is that is attacking you.

Your immune-producing "factories" are located in your bone marrow, lymph nodes, thymus (located at the front of your chest,) spleen and in the lymphoid tissues of your tonsils, adenoids and Peyer's patches (located in your intestinal system.) They are at work literally 24 hours a day, seven days a week. They do not stop. However, they do slow down when you sleep, which is good, because that is the only rest that they get (another reason for a good night's sleep). The reason that they are constantly working is that they had and still have poor union representation and were sold a bill of goods in the six days God was setting up shop here on earth. Apparently nobody told them that life would not be fair. Besides that unfortunate planning on their part, you are constantly getting bombarded by negative influences, which keeps the immune system on alert 24/7.

To aid the internal battle going on inside of your body, your immune system gladly welcomes the help (it certainly needs it) of outside mercenaries, whether or not they are getting paid for the services they will provide. (Of course, not having to pay for this help would be preferred.) These mercenaries come in the form of the antioxidants that you ingest either directly from the food you eat or the many supplements that you take. These kamikazes usually sacrifice themselves, killing the invading substance, or at least rendering them useless, thus eliminating your immune system from having to compensate them for their services. Life is tough in the mercenary business.

You can find antioxidants in most fruits and vegetables (assuming you don't cook them too long), herbs, teas, coffees, most vitamins and many other substances especially the ones naturally occurring in this world. *With all the negative stresses that your body is getting hit with on a consistent basis, you need the extra help of these invaluable mercenaries.* The additional benefit of making these a huge part of your diet is that they will, in turn make your immune system stronger which will make it all the more effective in its fight to keep you healthy.

THE EVIL AXIS

So whom are they fighting? Who is the dreaded enemy and can they be bribed or enticed? Substances that cause cancer and destroy cells are the main culprits, but they also have helpers. Single-celled creatures called bacteria, which are the smallest substance able to eat and reproduce by itself are not usually a problem. Your immune system seldom has difficulty with them, but in diseases like pneumonia, the shear numbers of invading bacteria are too much for your system to handle. A rather new phenomenon is the antibiotic-resistant bacteria. God help you if you run into one of these super-bacteria strains. These little bastards were born from the selective process of over-using antibiotic. Antibiotics kill most bacteria, but the ones that it doesn't kill, selectively get stronger and reproduce. The next antibiotic series wipes out a lot of them again, but the same thing happens. After a while, you have a huge colony that have a natural resistance to antibiotics and that's what causes the problem. By the way, many of these can be found residing in your favorite neighborhood hospital. Avoid antibiotics unless you absolutely need them!

In addition to antibiotic-resistant bacteria, discussed earlier, molds and yeasts are another category of the unseen creatures that wish to do you harm. Luckily, they aren't very good at it and are usually controllable. Viruses, found in most all of your cells, are parasites and are not capable of living on their own. So they'll just infect your cells and take them over. The little weasels! Also on your long list of enemies are poisons, toxins and other outside substance and chemicals. They would love to invade your body either through your nose, mouth and/or skin so as to tangle with your immune system. "Bring em on, we're ready."

What is the relationship of these cell-mutating antigens to your overall attitude about life? **The chemical changes that occur inside your body when you are ill are the same chemical reactions that happen when you are stressed, depressed, unhappy or just at an emotional low state for too long.** The same chemical changes translate into similar physical maladies.

Note the following symptoms that can be used to illustrate that you are ill and see if many of them also occur when you are not up to speed emotionally. Fever, memory loss, decreased appetite and thirst, reduction in physical activity, lack of interest in things that would normally would hold your attention, lack of assertiveness and energy in general and increased awareness to pain-all of these symptoms share a common denominator for both physical and emotional illness.

As important as all of the above-mentioned functions are to your life, they are nothing compared to the many subliminal ways your mind can assist you in reaching your goal of a long and healthy life. The human brain is the most powerful influence affecting mankind today. It always has and always will. It can truly be as powerful as you wish it to be. What a tool to have in your arsenal.

Cup of Tea

Is your cup half full or half empty? Be honest with yourself in assessing whether or not you are a positive or a negative person, an optimist or a pessimist. No one is happy or upbeat all of the time.

There has to be balance in your life, since there is no such thing as a real life Pollyanna.

So, how do you fit in, overall? Do you look for the brighter things in life or is someone always out to get you? Do you see the best in people or are you so concerned with how they compare to you that you fail to see them as they truly are? And why are we asking such personal questions?

Your outlook on life and your overall attitude can literally affect the quality and length of time you reside on this earth. **There are tons of research pointing to the powers of the human brain and how it affects your overall health and well-being.** These effects can be tracked and measured by actual physical changes within your system, usually through an increase or decrease in your immune function. (One of the ways to compute the effectiveness of your immune system is to gauge the amount of immunoglobulin, a disease fighter residing in you saliva. It is quite simple to measure and is usually done before and after the study being conducted.)

Stormin' Norman

In 1964, Norman Cousins the long-time editor of *Saturday Review* was diagnosed with, among other things, ankylosing spondylitis, at the time, a debilitating collagen disease that attacks the connective tissues of virtually every cell in your body, but concentrates in the joint areas especially the spinal cord. (All arthritic and rheumatic diseases fall into this category.) He was unable to lie down comfortably, turn over, use any of his limbs and he certainly couldn't get up without extreme pain. Cousins was basically in a world of hurt and was living on massive painkillers. He turned down radiation and chemotherapy treatments, a good move. In fact, his doctors told him to get his life in order- he had three months to live. He was thirty-nine years old.

Mr. Cousins didn't accept this verdict, and it's a good thing that he didn't. He lived to be seventy-five, outlasting his prognosis by thirty-six years. Did medical science cure him? Not quite. In fact, it would have killed him if he hadn't done two things. **First, he grabbed away the control of his care and took his future into his own hands,** and second he tried a couple of "treatments" that not only were considered radical for the time, but also were unheard of.

What did he do? Well, to make a long story somewhat shorter, he first analyzed why he caught this seemingly deadly disease. He correctly decided that his immune system had failed him on an exhaustive trip to Moscow and the diesel fumes he had been constantly breathing in from the open windows of his hotel while there had doomed him. His immune system, notably his endocrine and adrenal functions, had collapsed and left him defenseless to fight off any illness. He just happened to be unlucky enough to contract this horribly uncomfortable, and quite possibly deadly, disease.

He remembered reading several years earlier that stress, emotional tension, and suppressed rage, among other negative emotional behaviors could literally trash one's immune system; he wondered if the opposite were true. What would positive emotions do to his disease-fighting system? Since the negative end of the behavior spectrum changed body chemistry for the worse, would positive behavior alter it for the better?

One thing that helped him was that he had a doctor who realized that modern medicine (in 1964) was still clueless to many of the illnesses that plagued mankind (still are, judging by the number of diseases that are killing more and more Americans than ever before) and he was open to any possible solution that might work. Norman's arguments were apparently convincing enough to get him to go along with this virtual self-treatment. So he moved out of the hospital and into a hotel nearby.

The first thing addressed was his medication. **The aspirin and the phenylbutazone they were giving him were justifiable for their anti-inflammatory and painkilling characteristics, but he suspected (correctly) that they were toxic to his system and he stopped using them immediately.** Their side effects would have been enough to convince him that they were causing large, competing problems all by themselves.

He also read about the curative effects of ascorbic acid (vitamin C) on several ailments and diseases and decided to try massive doses in a drip I.V. as his first and only chemical action. No medicine, no painkillers, no nothing but nutrients, fluids and vitamin C. But then there was the pain. For that, he decided to test his positive emotional-behavior theory and brought in every funny movie he could find. Today, that would be easy, but in 1964 there were no VCRs, DVDs, ISDN, etc. However, lucky for him, he was connected with the media and was able to get a projector and plenty of films like *Candid Camera,* the Marx Brothers and Abbott and Costello. Anything he could find that was funny, he watched. Every time the pain was becoming unbearable, he would have a good belly laugh and an amazing thing happened. His level of pain diminished and he began to improve.

You might think that this was a very subjective response, but he tested it scientifically. There is a test called a "sed-rate," a blood test measuring the rate that your red blood cells settle in a test tube measured in millimeters per hour. This corresponds directly with the level of inflammation. The higher the number, the sicker you are. A slight illness would have a sed-rate of about thirty to forty. Sixty to seventy was a real problem. Cousins' sed-rate was well over one hundred! Every time he watched funny movies, his sed-rate dropped significantly and continued to slowly drop over time as long as he used this type of treatment. **He actually documented the positive change in body chemistry from having pleasurable feelings!**

It took several months to get back into his routine, and it was years before he was totally back to normal as far as joint flexibility and comfort go, but the point is that he beat it. He beat the medical establishment, but more importantly he cured himself with nothing more than some vitamin C and some good laughs. Not bad, huh? By the way, he stated that he had "a fast-growing conviction that a hospital is no place for a person who is *seriously* ill." He was an astute man truly ahead of his time. This is but one example of the power of that globe being balanced on the top of your shoulders. There are more . . . several more.

"After not feeling well for some time, a guy goes to his doctor who tells him that he has six months to live. In five months, he goes back in and tells the doc that he doesn't have enough to pay his bill, so the doctor gives him six more months to live."

"My friend, upon seeing his troubling chest x-rays from his annual checkup, told his doctor that he would pay him extra to touch them up."

"There were two blondes who went deep into the frozen woods searching for a Christmas tree. After hours of sub-zero temperatures, a few close calls with hungry wolves, one blonde turned to the other and said, 'I'm chopping down the next tree I see. I don't care whether it's decorated or not!'"

"When I read about the evils of drinking, I gave up reading."

"If Wal-mart is lowering prices every day, how come nothing in the store is free yet?"

O.K. At least chuckle . . . There, you just lengthened your life by a nano-second.

Show me

Way back in prehistoric times, around the 1940s, a group of Harvard grads were given an attitudinal questionnaire to determine their degree of optimism or pessimism. A trio of researchers then tracked the study group every five years and found an interesting correlation between the two different degrees of behavior. Between the ages of forty and forty-five, the optimists began showing physical signs of being healthier than the pessimists, indicating that your attitude can influence your overall health.

Further, Christopher Peterson, Ph.D. from the University of Michigan, a pioneer in the field of psychology and its relation to health and one of the researchers in the above-mentioned study also determined that pessimists tend to be ill and miss work more often than optimists.

Dr. Martin Seligman, who wrote *Authentic Happiness,* says that optimists are happier, have healthier habits and eventually live longer because they have lower blood pressure and stronger immune systems. (By the way, he also found that they are more productive at work and hence are paid more, plus an interesting observation is that they tend to view any misfortune as temporary.) The implication here is that things don't get them down for too terribly long and that, by itself, keeps them healthy.

The bottom line is that the better you feel about yourself, the better your outlook is concerning your life and the better your overall attitude, the healthier you will be. Now, is your cup half full yet? If not, run to the kitchen and fill it up!

Humor and attitude are not the only psychological characteristics that can affect your well-being. Can you use direct manipulation of your thoughts to affect your physical condition? One study demonstrating the power of meditation used a disease that would be readily observable and not left to subjectivity. Eczema, a sometimes hideous-looking skin disorder was cleared up 40% quicker by adding only a mantra that the patients used in addition to the light therapy and medication that all of the participants received. The mantra was nothing more than reassuring positive statements that you would use if you were trying to talk yourself into feeling better.

The food connection

There are many different types of foods that help keep your brain healthy including many vitamin-rich fruits and vegetables and essential fatty acids. If, however you still don't believe there is any relationship between what you eat and how it affects the way you think, then think again.

Research has shown a link between the overall amount of, and the type of fatty acids consumed in a country and the level of depression reported in that nation. Countries with the highest consumption of fish also have the lowest rate of depression. What you eat *does* have some degree of control over how long you live.

Take two placebos and call me in the morning

You have certainly heard of "the placebo effect," a term used to balance studies and research on a particular cure or effects of drugs, supplements or any other substance on the human body. A placebo could very well be a sham surgery, a shot, I.V. or anything else. For our explanation, please envision a placebo as a sugar pill used instead of a pharmaceutical, both given in the same manner with the only variable in the study being the difference in the pills. (In a double-blind study, the subjects are usually divided in half and then administered the substance. They know that they are in a study, but don't know if they are getting the drug or the placebo and neither do the people administering the dosage, thus the double-blind aspect of the experiment). In virtually every study, people on the placebo seem to receive at least some benefit from the treatment even though there was nothing in the pill other than sugar water.

Isn't the placebo effect the perfect example of the power of your mind? Even if you don't understand why it worked, the fact that it did is nothing short of amazing. Generally speaking, anywhere from 20 to 60% of the subjects, sometimes more, receiving the sugar pill get at least some relief from . . . nothing. Given that fact, where is the relief coming from?

What has happened in every case of placebo use is that in the patients' mind, they believe that they are going to get better, whether it's from nothing more than the doctor saying that they will, or from the pill that they think is going to help them. That belief and the power of the human brain have actually changed the body's chemistry for its host's benefit. **Whether it was a surgery not performed, a drug or supplement not given or a therapy not done normally, the absolute power of the human brain took control of the healing process by itself.** You could say that the placebo gave some amount of relief all on its own.

There have been several studies involving placebo surgeries that have all shown that the sham surgery was at least as beneficial as the actual, supposedly corrective surgery! These are truly amazing. One study was conducted on older Americans who had bum knees. Half of them had the actual surgery, the other half had their knees cut open, but then sewn right back up. **Those with the placebo surgery recovered quicker and more completely than the ones with the actual corrective procedure.** How do we explain that?

There have been several other sham surgeries done, all above board and for study purposes, that have continuously shown a reduction in pain. A small study in Houston where an orthopedic surgeon operated on ten knees by making an incision only and performing no work on the knees at all was apparently a complete success. All ten of the patients felt much better. (I hope that they didn't have to pay for the surgeries that they didn't actually receive!)

Another study in Seattle was conducted on people with acute angina (pains in the chest area.) A cardiologist operated on them to relieve the pain, but all he did was to make an incision in their chests and then sew them back up. Even though they knew that they were part of a study, 90% of them said they felt better and had less chest pains than before the sham surgery. Amazing.

Now, obviously, if you have an 80% blockage of the blood flow to your heart, or you have broken your leg, being told that you're going to get better by itself isn't going to fix the problem. Your brain isn't that talented. You will need the actual surgery. However, in areas dealing with levels of discomfort, pain and immune functions, the placebo has shown that your brain is a very powerful tool that should be used in maintaining your vitality.

We tend to look at the placebo effect entirely in the wrong context. A recent study involving St. John's Wort showed that it didn't have much better results in curbing mild depression than the placebo. Although this particular study was flawed at best, the fact that the placebo had any affect at all is tremendous. Instead of condemning the product being tested, salute the power of your mind and its ability to heal you. Recognize that it is very powerful and learn to use it to your benefit. Start by telling yourself that your neighbor is not really a jerk, but is a jewel of a person. Doesn't that make you feel better?

HAVE FAITH!

You've been told since you were a child that going to church on a regular basis was good for your soul. It turns out that, not only is it good for your soul, it's not bad for your immune system either. Any kind of faith and specifically prayer has been shown in several studies to have absolute benefit to your health. People who do are healthier and live longer than people who don't.

Duke University sponsored a study that monitored 4000 older men and women of all faiths and found that the risk of dying was 46% lower in those who went to religious services on a regular basis. Of the same study, those who prayed regularly also had much lower blood pressure levels than those who didn't.

Other studies demonstrated healthier immune systems, better surgery survival rates, and speedier recovery from depression, alcoholism, drug addiction, arthritis and heart attacks from having faith. Surviving AIDS patients did so more often through religious faith than those who didn't have any faith.

Scientists aren't exactly sure why prayer and religious conviction keep you healthy, but they have noticed a couple of documented physical changes in the human body. One of those changes was shown to occur by Dr. Andy Newberg, the author of *Why God Won't Go Away* who noted changes in blood flow to specific regions of the brain during times of prayer. He also notes the observance of lower blood pressure, decreased anxiety and a better sense of well-being.

Prayer and faith are garnishing a lot of attention today in the medical community as they pertain to your overall health. Some physicians are even including them as a part of their treatment. Dr. Larry Dossey, the author of *Healing Words* and *Prayer is Good Medicine* said, "I decided that not using prayer on behalf of my patients was the equivalent of withholding a needed medication or surgical procedure."

While on this subject, no evidence has been shown that praying for others can help them unless you happen to be in their presence. Praying near to them could very well lift their spirits and give them a feeling of belonging and acceptance. Praying for people certainly can't hurt them and very well may help you, but several studies have failed to show a positive relationship while not in their presence. That's not to say that future studies won't show different results . . . unless you're praying for the Chicago Cubs. Sadly, there is no hope for them.

YOU CAN PICK YOUR FRIENDS AND YOU CAN PICK YOUR...

Since we have established that good, positive and pleasurable experiences can all boost your immune system, it makes sense that the friends that you keep and the people with whom you associate can influence your health, too. People sometimes complain that they don't have any control in their lives. Well, choosing your friends is one area where you do have control. Other than the people that you work with, when you punch the time clock on your way out the door, you control who you phone, who you visit and whose party you'll attend this coming weekend.

According to Dr.'s Francis Brennan and Carl Charnetski who co-wrote the book, *Feeling Good is Good for You,* they recommend being around people who are funny, optimistic and good conversationalists. Don't hang around those who need to be in total control of their surroundings. People that like you just because they like being around you and not because of some power trip they are on are a lot better for your well-being.

Also, everyone has at least one friend who is self-destructive by nature. You know the ones we're talking about. They build themselves up only to crash and burn at the bottom and then begin building themselves up again. So much wasted potential and such a waste of energy, it's a shame that they do this to themselves. You do not need to jump onto their roller coaster for obvious reasons, unless you like being around those who have it worse than you. Don't be their psychologist.

SWEAT IT OUT

Exercise has been proven to have a positive affect on your immune system. This is accomplished in several ways. People who exercise on a regular basis feel better about themselves, feel better about how they look and maybe the weight that they have lost.

They feel like they have accomplished something, done something for themselves and nobody else. Their self-esteem is boosted just by the effort that they have made at the gym, contributing to the many emotional benefits of exercise without even mentioning any of the physical attributes.

Exercise lowers your blood pressure and your resting heart-rate, it releases serotonin which helps you relax and inhibits the release of the immune-killing chemical called cortisol. Being a regular gym rat increases your muscle mass while decreasing the amount of fat you are carrying, especially the dangerous kind around your mid-section. It halts osteoporosis, drives toxins out of your system, increases the efficiency of your organs and can improve your sex life . . . if you have one. Getting a good night's sleep is also easier with exercise. Every single one of the above-mentioned benefits of exercise helps your immune system too, so please begin a regular exercise program if you haven't already.

Other than getting hit by a car while jogging, the only negative aspect of exercise as it relates to your immune system is if you overdo it. If you are a world-class marathoner or tri-athlete logging dozens of hours of strenuous exercising weekly, you may be compromising your immune system. There is a diminishing rate of return as exercise pertains to your immune function, but I doubt seriously if any of us have that problem, so keep working at it.

Spread it around

How many of you would love to work in a chocolate factory? How about inside a Domino's Pizza restaurant? For you chocolate and pizza freaks, that may sound like a wonderfully satisfying career move, but you know that after a while you would get sick of even smelling the food. There is a biological reason to go along with the psychological one. A little chocolate (preferably dark chocolate) is actually good for you and your body recognizes that by pumping out pleasure-inducing peptides when you partake, which in turn stimulates your immune system. After a while, your brain quits producing them. In other words, "I've had enough," says your brain! "Let's move onto something else, like collard greens!" It doesn't require a lot of these rich foods to get the nutrition it is looking for and it lets you know when it has had enough, if you will listen.

Likewise, in the foods you eat, a little goes a long way for many, many reasons, one of them being for your immune system. Take in a little chocolate here, a little coffee there and some funny movies . . . occasionally. Sit through all of *The Pink Panther* movies in one day and its doubtful that you'll get the benefit of much more than watching just one of them. Moderation allows you to keep your mind active, allows you to experience many different things and will maximize your potential for helping out your poor, overworked immune system.

VENTILATE

How well do you do with pent-up aggression? Do you keep everything bottled up inside or do you blow an internal gasket when things get to be too much? You probably have guessed that neither response is good for you or your immune system. Several studies over the years have shown that both responses can suppress your immune function and compromise your health. Plus, **people that appear okay on the outside and even state that all is fine when it is not, have the same immune problems of the volatile and repressive people mentioned above.**

So, what is the proper response to negative and stressful emotions? Regularly talking to someone about your problems, whether it be a counselor, close friend, clergy, family member or even the guy sitting next to you on the commuter train seems to be the best way to vent out your frustrations and concerns without negatively impacting your immune function, and in the long run, your life. Everyone needs someone to talk to . . . sounds like a country western song. Nonetheless, slowly letting the steam out of your system is better for you than either blowing or seething. Besides, blowing up at the wrong time in front of the wrong person could be bad for your immediate health, especially if the person you are blowing at is bigger than you and is also looking for someone to rip apart! However, buying a punching bag and getting a workout while venting some anger kills two birds at the same time. It's much cheaper than starting your own demolition derby in the supermarket parking lot.

A FINAL WORD

There are many examples of the ways your brain and your overall attitude influences your immune system, and in the long run, the time you spend above the topsoil. The major theme to remember is that most any positive emotion is a lot better for you than the opposite. Being happy, content, amused, rewarded, tickled, well adjusted, serene and comfortable benefit you. Being well rested, full of energy, having feelings of vitality and being on top of the world will also do wonders for you. Listening to good music, being entertained by a funny movie, having a good workout, and maybe a good cry can all be beneficial. Seeing the good in people and finding that half-full cup may help you to live longer. The next time you begin to let negative thoughts into your head, remember that they can hurt you and keep you from your goal of a long and happy life. Here's to you and your beautiful mind! Now, go fill *all* of your cups completely to the top.

Step 10:

Alternative Therapies

Hopefully, by now, we have established that the western medical community, in general, does not have all the answers when it comes to your health. Not only are they not in the business to prevent diseases before they happen, they are unable to manage or cure many of them once you are unlucky enough to contract one. Western medicine's curative bag of goodies include masking pain through prescription drugs, relieving symptoms through prescription drugs, using prescription drugs to wipe out many of your functioning systems and healthy cells (through radiation and chemotherapy) while hopefully taking the disease with it (kind of like Napalm), using non-selective prescription antibiotics that kill most of the bacteria in your system including the beneficial ones, and occasionally curing the disease, of course while using prescription drugs, without doing too much damage to the rest of your body. In other words, "you'll live."

STOP! We are tired of this! Why did the disease enter your body in the first place? You ate at the same places, worked in similar jobs, lived in the same neighborhood and had the same basic lifestyle as everyone you know, so why did disease pick on you? Ever had that question answered by a doctor? Probably not, nor were you given advice on how to keep disease from paying you a visit in the first place. That should be what medicine is all about. Live healthy and give your body what it needs and you will remain healthy. Have a strong immune system; don't get sick and then react to it by obtaining drugs to try and fix the problem. Prevent disease before it strikes.

Most alternative therapies don't involve the use of prescription drugs to react to disease, they use methods to enhance your immune system, build up your body's strength, allowing it to do the job it was designed to do, which is to heal you from within. **They use techniques to relieve pain, lower stress and relax you, with the knowledge that your body will not be able to take proper care of itself while there is pain, discomfort, or disease.** Remove these obstacles and the greatest invention the world will ever see, the human body, will take over the task and succeed in slaying whatever it is that is trying to take you down. Again, if given the chance, your body will heal itself.

Supplements have gone mainstream, so they aren't included in this section. There are many herbs taken internally that can do a world of good and some were covered previously. The following practices, although incomplete, constitute a good sampling of what is considered alternative medicine. If you have found a type of healing that you like and isn't mentioned here, wonderful! If it works for you, then keep on using it, if not, maybe some of these may help.

This section isn't a complete guide for all alternative therapies. It is meant to merely show some of many different options that you have at your disposal, if you are not getting all that you need or desire presently from the world of healthcare.

CHIROPRACTIC

Chiro, the Greek word for hand, and practic, meaning practice or operation. A chiropractor's primary job is to determine the presence of nerve interference. Then, he (or she) manipulates the spine to help the body put itself in a position to correct itself. If the spine is out of alignment, then the flow of energy through the nerves is disrupted; this being the chiropractor's basis for treating many ailments and discomforts.

Today's form of chiropractic care began in the mid 1890s by a D.D. Palmer and was furthered by his son, B.J. Palmer who developed the philosophy and science of the practice that we now know. However, spinal manipulation, which is the basis for this practice, had its start eons ago. The Chinese were using it in 2700 B.C., the Greeks, a little different version in 1500 B.C. The ancient Egyptians, Babylonians, Hindus, Tibetans, and Syrians all practiced some form of spinal manipulation. Hippocrates, considered the father of medicine was a big proponent of manipulation of the spine. He stated, "Get knowledge of the spine, for this is the requisite for many diseases."

Today's chiropractor is as regulated and schooled as most medical doctors. They are licensed by every state. Each of the colleges require as many hours of study as a medical doctor and the facilities that the schools use have given them thousands of hours of clinical of experience.

Whether you believe in chiropractic or not, you must be aware that the human back literally takes a beating over time as a result of everything from gravity and improper lifting, to a wrong sleep position and even stress; it is only logical that it can get slightly misaligned from time to time. After x-raying your back, a chiropractor will attempt to gently nudge the misaligned vertebrae back to where it is supposed to be, freeing the flow of nerve signals from your brain and restoring the proper balance to your system.

This will allow your body's *innate intelligence,* as it is referred to in chiropractic vernacular, to take care of any ailments you may be suffering from.

Innate intelligence is abundant in every living being, whether it is a plant, animal, or microorganism on this planet. It guides its host in all facets of life, from causing a plant to turn towards the sun for its energy, to your body properly reacting to a cut on your arm. Something tells your brain that there is a problem through the pain or discomfort that you felt from the cut, rushes your microbe-fighting blood cells to the area to fortify its defenses, sends clotting instructions to the area to keep you from bleeding to death and then tells you to look for sympathy from your loved one so that they will kiss it and make it all better. This is but one example of the absolutely remarkable machine called the human body; there are literally millions more.

Call it what you may, but without this innate intelligence, we would not be here today. It makes perfect sense that if you disrupt the nerve flow in your body, you will have a host of varied problems, ranging from pain and discomfort in your limbs and back, to chronic fatigue and headaches. Problems such as asthma, sinus problems, allergies, poor posture, constipation, arthritis, pain in less obvious joints, foot problems, irritability and a lack of concentration, are but a few of the ailments that chiropractic may help by improving that energy flow through your spine.

Acupuncture and acupressure refer to this form of energy as chi ("chee," not as in chi tea at Starbucks). With chiropractors, it is innate intelligence. Regardless of how you refer to it as, there is much to be learned about the human body, its relationship with bio-electrical energy and how that correlates with you biological functions. This is one of those areas that we know little about. However, there has been some work done in this field.

Dr. Robert Becker, in his book, *The Body Electric,* explains the flow of electrical energy throughout the human body. He actually mapped out verifiable electrical juncture points that correspond almost exactly to the pressure points used in acupuncture and acupressure hopefully lending western legitimacy to these tried and true therapies. Dr. Becker and others have demonstrated how certain types of electrical currents can not only heal wounds quicker, but even allows the regeneration of fingertips that have been severed! The 21st century should see remarkable work done in this field. Until then, don't dismiss chiropractic or the Chinese practices as quackery. You may not understand them, but know that many times they can work wonders.

As far as chiropractic goes, if you have been diagnosed with an actual protruding disc, a broken bone in your back, or any other major spine problem, an orthopedic or neurological doctor should be your first contact.

When visiting a chiropractor, the last thing that you will get is a prescription drug. Preventative care is as big apart of their practice as is manipulation, and for that reason the right chiropractor may be able to help you immensely.

Osteopathic Medicine

Mate a medical doctor with a chiropractor (they should preferably be of the opposite sex) and the result would be a baby osteopath, not to be confused with a baby psychopath. An osteopathic doctor is basically a primary medical doctor with an advanced knowledge of the human musculoskeletal system. They can prescribe medicine, if they must, but as with chiropractors, they believe that the human body is more than just the sum of the parts. They realize that all systems of the human body are connected in some form, and to treat only one specific problem without looking at the overall human being attached to that problem would not serve their patient properly. They also believe in preventative care as a proactive approach to health instead of a reactive response as it pertains to disease.

An osteopathic doctor (a D.O. instead of M.D.) has the same basic training as a general practitioner with the above-mentioned extra training in the musculoskeletal system and, when needed, they adjust the spine as a chiropractor would.

As with medical doctors, osteopaths complete four years of medical school, they both must pass comparable state licensing exams, they both practice in licensed and accredited health-care facilities, but osteopaths are encouraged to be primary care physicians focusing on preventative health care. You probably won't find too many neurological surgeons that are D.O.s, but if you were cared for by an osteopath, you might not need one.

If you have the choice (osteopaths are usually an acceptable option with insurance companies) between a M.D. and a D. O., and you don't have any severe, specific problems like a failing heart, then a Doctor of Osteopathic Medicine may be an excellent choice for a general physician. At least you know that preventative medicine is a priority to them and prescription drugs are not.

Rolfing

Have you been Rolfed today? That's what I thought. Neither have I! Besides the sheer fun of saying the word, "Rolfing," this technique has become popular while gaining many followers over the last half century. Dr. Ida Rolf developed and began using this technique over fifty years ago. Referred to as *Structural Integration,* this technique generally utilizes strong, soft tissue manipulation (muscles and connective tissues) to re-organize the structure of the spine and surrounding areas with the intent to de-constrict and re-balance the body. In the way this is accomplished, it is similar in theory to the chiropractic therapy; the main difference being in the manipulation of the muscles and connective fascia instead of the bones themselves. Having a Rolfing session (there are ten in the initial program) is like getting a strong massage . . . a really strong one. So hard that the practitioners, over time, developed a much softer method to appease us wimps!

This practice, although fairly new in relation to many other alternative therapies, is quite popular. Everyone likes a good massage, and this is one of the best that you can get, if you can stand the relative discomfort of some of the techniques. The main difference between this and a regular massage, besides the intensity, has to do with the plan or direction the Rolfing practitioner is following. Not only are they massaging the muscles in general, they are attempting to manipulate certain tissues in a specific way as to loosen up parts of the spine. Now, go get Rolfed.

HOMEOPATHY

The practice of homeopathy was re-discovered and named by a German doctor, Samuel Hahnemann in the early 1800s. He identified the modern principle of homeopathy while experimenting on himself in an effort to better understand how some medicines of his time worked. Being dissatisfied with the typical treatments used, like blood-letting, leeches, and medicines that oftentimes caused more damage than the disease it was trying to cure such as mercury and lead cleansings, he questioned the entire basis of why these treatments were used in the first place. While translating a text on the use of quinine as a treatment for malaria, he wondered how its use would affect a healthy person, so, like any good scientist, he consumed Cinchona bark, which is used to make quinine. After several days, he experienced the symptoms of malaria, which continued until he stopped taking the quinine concoction. Thus his theory of "like curing like" evolved.

I'll admit that homeopathy is a very difficult concept to comprehend. It is based on a principle of "similars," which means that anything that makes you ill can also cure you. If a healthy person chewed on basil for several days and eventually experienced the symptoms of hay fever, then the basil should cure a person actually suffering from the ailment, which, according to believers in homeopathy, it does. Thus, the principle of similars.

Many of the homeopathic cures are difficult to prove scientifically, so you can imagine the degree of skepticism cast upon it by the medical profession. However, it continues to work in many people and that is why it has lasted for two hundred years. Modern medicine is based on antidotes, or opposite medicines and it's not hard to understand why our medical society has a problem with it. Having acid stomach problems? Prescribe a "base," at the opposite end of the pH spectrum to cure the problem. Homeopathy might suggest using an acid to correct the problem.

One of the many reasons that our western medical community has such a problem with homeopathy is that, for it to be effective, it must be diluted so extensively that the original ingredient is no longer recognizable. Practitioners believe that the more diluted the liquid, the more potent it actually becomes. So a 6x solution is not as effective as a 12x, the number denoting the number of times the solution has been diluted.

Proponents would argue that not only does conventional medicine still use a variety of drugs that have been shown to be effective by trial and error only such as many anti-depressants, but vaccines themselves are very similar in the way that they both work. Another argument could be said for taking a small dose of aspirin to prevent a heart attack, where as a much larger dose would not be advisable. Very strange, but who can argue with results?

Regardless what you think about homeopathy, it is generally very safe because of the level of dilution and it may be worth a try on problems such as sinusitis, headaches, chronic fatigue, stress, insomnia, stomach and digestive ailments, arthritis and acne.

Obviously, if you have a broken leg, severe heart problems or a tumor protruding from the side of your head, you had better leave those and any other major problem to a medical doctor. For ailments that are symptomatic in nature that are somewhat controlled by Western medicine without actually being cured, then homeopathy may be worth a try.

Naturopathic Medicine

This is more of a philosophical approach to good health and well being than any specific form of medicine. As the name implies, a naturopath will lean toward a more natural and less-invasive form of preventative care to keep the body healthy rather than a pharmaceutical drug given after disease has struck. My kind of doctor! A naturopath may be a medical doctor; yet he or she doesn't have to be to give dietary and lifestyle advice.

Many of the recommendations a naturopath might impart will be many of the same suggestions given in this program. A plant-based diet, a moderate level of exercise, the proper supplementation of herbs, minerals and vitamins, stress reduction and lifestyle changes are all tools in the naturopath's bag. Unfortunately they sometimes recommend things like colonic cleanses and other detoxifying routines that are suspect at best, and possibly dangerous. Some swear by these type of treatments, but it would be irresponsible to recommend them here.

A naturopath has many, many wonderful treatments to recommend and some to stay clear of. Use your common sense and you will make the right decision.

Aromatherapy

There is not any form of medicine or therapy of any kind that is older than aromatherapy. It began thousands of years ago with the ancient Egyptians, who extracted essential oils from aromatic plants to be used in medicines and cosmetics. Around the same time, the Chinese also were experimenting with oils for medicinal purposes, but took it a step further and burned the oils with wood in a show of respect for their gods. This particular practice is still used today. The Greeks furthered the investigation into the uses of essential oils and passed their knowledge onto the Romans who were well known for their scented baths and massages that followed. (Sounds like a great idea, right about now!) Unfortunately, aromatherapy and just about everything else of any therapeutic value died out during the European dark ages...if only they would have bathed a little more often!

Today has shown the resurgence in aromatherapy with the increased awareness of the connection of mind and body and how they can work together to bring about better health, which is one reason to support this practice.

Aromatherapy is the use of essential oils extracted from aromatic plants to enhance health, well being and beauty. (Tough to argue with.) The essential oils are very volatile oils that are actually essential to the particular plant's survival and are extracted by distillation, expression, or the use of solvents. If the solvent method is used, the solvent must be totally extracted from the compound leaving only the concentrated oil. The oils usually cannot be used in their concentrated form. They must be diluted tremendously, unless you like a receiving a nasty burn or extremely uncomfortable irritation. A few drops per use are generally all that is required, but you should defer to the instructions of the particular oil for proper usage.

You're probably already practicing some form of aromatherapy by burning scented candles, using cough drops, pine oil cleaners or antiseptic mouthwashes. They are used as a base in many products that you use around the house. Just don't admit to your doctor that you are using them for medicinal purposes or he may have you committed. Essential oils have been around for a long time, but apparently not long enough to secure the blessings of the Western medical community.

As in homeopathy, don't count on essential oils to cure you of cancer, but they have, and can have many uses in your journey to find and remain healthy. You've already learned about the power of your mind and the devastating effects of stress and how they both affect your overall level of health. Aromatherapy can assist both of these and is a valuable tool for you to use to make your life easier. By using eucalyptus oil for colds and the flu, ginger to relax your digestive muscles, chamomile to calm down or basil for your sinuses, your overall health can be improved without a whole lot of interference in your day-to-day life. Aromatherapy is a real winner.

You can actually have a lot of fun with this extremely old therapy by adding essential oils to your bath, lotions, candle wax, pot-pourri and morning cereal. (Nix that last one.) Your sources of specific information on aromatherapy include many books, health food stores, gift and candle shops, the internet and several health magazines.

Acupuncture

Acupuncture, one of the several therapies that constitute traditional Chinese medicine has in fact, gone mainstream. The National Institute of Health has concluded that acupuncture indeed does alleviate nausea and pain and may be effective in treating a host of other discomforts and ailments. There are over 10,000 registered, licensed and/or certified acupuncturists operating in the United States. In addition, over 3,000 medical doctors or doctors of osteopath also practice here. Long gone are the days of considering it a form of voodoo medicine, arbitrarily sticking patients with long, jagged needles.

The Chinese believe that the body, mind and soul all work together to bring harmony to the entire being. Acupuncture works by restoring this flow of chi (sometimes spelled "Qi"), the life force that is involved in all bodily functions. They believe chi travels along fourteen channels, or meridians, on each side of the body, surfacing at approximately 360 points. These points are where the needles are then inserted. These needles are sometimes stimulated by rotating the needles, heating with a scented flame or by using a small and safe level of electrical stimulation to enhance the affect. The sessions normally last twenty to thirty minutes.

My first visual experience with acupuncture was several years ago while viewing a brain surgery being performed on a fully conscious Chinese woman. This PBS special narrated by Leonard Nimoy, of *Star Trek* fame, showed the top of this patient's head being opened up like a cookie jar, the only form of anesthesia used was four acupuncture needles strategically placed and then stimulated by an electric current. The patient stated that she could feel the vibration of the surgical skill-saw used to open her up, but no discomfort. (The doctors kept her conscious so as to observe her reactions to the probing of her brain. They needed to do so for the success of this particular surgery.)

Dr. Isadore Rosentheld, who writes for *Parade Magazine,* took a photo of a twenty-eight year-old patient having open-heart surgery performed at the University of Shanghai in the mid 1980s. If he hadn't witnessed this event, he may not have believed that the only form of anesthesia being used for this surgery was a single electrically stimulated needle inserted in the patient's right earlobe. She was wide-awake while her chest was wide open! I think it is safe to assume that acupuncture may, just may reduce pain!

Will it work for you? Again, if your arm is broken, your heart has stopped beating or you're spitting up blood, then stick to conventional medicine. If you suffer from: headaches, heartburn, chronic fatigue, back and neck pain, sinusitis, arthritis, asthma or similar types of problems, acupuncture may very well help alleviate the discomfort. Any problem involving chronic pain or discomfort, long-term suffering or just constant misery may be helped by acupuncture.

The majority of states require some form of certification or license to practice acupuncture. The educational requirements vary from a low of 1,300 up to 2,600 hours of training by an accredited school and you should look for someone along that caliber. There are several sources of information and organizations that should help point you in the right direction. Please refer to the appendix for some of these. There are also many, many publications dealing with the entire field of acupuncture and are readily available at your library, bookstores, and through online bookstores like Amazon.com.

REFLEXOLOGY

Do you like to have your feet rubbed? If so, then you'll probably enjoy the work of a reflexologist. They believe that the feet have various reflex points connected to the rest of human body that are capable of relieving many stress-related problems, headaches, asthma, digestive problems, many forms of chronic pain and even some neurological disorders. There is some research to support some of these claims like headaches, but they lack clinical testing results to back the majority of claims.

Reflexology is closer to acupressure than massage in that the practitioner presses on the reflex point rather than massaging the foot. However, if you ask, they are sure to comply with your request!

BIOFEEDBACK

No machines for you to purchase, no expensive supplements or prescriptions to swallow, and nothing that can be patented and thus profited from, biofeedback is certainly on that proverbial island by itself. You don't hear a lot about this therapy because there isn't big money behind it. It may be the greatest thing in the world, but if the medical industry can't profit from it, you ain't gonna hear about it.

This seemingly unorthodox therapy probably won't cure you of cancer, but it can help to relieve many areas of discomfort and lessen symptoms in others. Biofeedback can help alleviate the ravages of arthritis, control high blood pressure, lessen depression, headaches, chronic fatigue syndrome, muscle spasms and can even control many digestive disorders like ulcers, chronic constipation, and irritable bowel syndrome.

How does it work? After being connected to several different pieces of equipment that measure everything from a change in body temperature to brain activity, a trained therapist will first demonstrate what the sensors show while you are experiencing different symptoms, whether or not you are aware of them, and then will teach you mental and physical exercises that will train you to control those bodily functions that are causing the problem. (Several sessions are usually required because of the difficulty of sensing and changing involuntary behaviors.)

Some of the equipment used are *skin temperature gauges* that actually show the change in blood flow, and of course, minute temperature changes, *electromyographs* (EMGs) that measure muscle tension, and *electroencephalographs* (EEGs) that measure brain waves. Also incorporated into this therapy are *electrocardiographs* (ECGs) that monitor heart rate, *galvanic skin response sensors* that measure the amount of sweat you produce under stress, and *respiration feedback* devices that monitor breathing cycles.

Biofeedback is a classic example of mind over matter demonstrating the sheer power of the human brain. If there was any doubt that the human brain has the ability to affect what goes on in the rest of the body, biofeedback puts those uncertainties to rest. If you partake, you will be shown in black and white by the little equipment monitors you are viewing the affect you are having on your body's actions.

It's not an easy, laidback experience. You will have to work for this control. This process can be physically and emotionally taxing as you train yourself to control whatever symptom it is that you are having problems with. You are dealing with normally involuntary functions and are attempting to control those.

Although this may not shrink tumors or clear up a bad x-ray, biofeedback can alleviate many, many uncomfortable ailments and disorders and since there are few, if any, side effects, it is certainly worth a try. Once you learn the control, your sessions should move to more of a maintenance mode and the frequency of them diminished.

CHELATION

Chelation therapy involves the injection of a chemical called ethylenediaminetetraacetic acid (we may want to call it EDTA) through an IV needle with the intent of removing excess amounts of metals from your system. Each treatment takes about three to four hours to complete and it is recommend to have anywhere from twenty to fifty treatments for it to be effective. This does not sound like a great idea unless you have been diagnosed with some sort of metal poisoning like lead, iron or aluminum, which it is effective against.

Its advocates claim that it can be used successfully against Alzheimer's, Multiple Sclerosis, Parkinson's, arthritis, psoriasis, thyroid problems, cancer and bad manners. They also claim that it boosts energy, prevents strokes, and improves mental awareness. (If it actually removed those excess metals from your system, then this would make sense). Maybe so, but there are way too many skeptics to trust this procedure.

Injecting a foreign substance into your veins, by itself, doesn't make sense. There are much better choices to cleanse your system and this program has outlined many of them, like a change in diet, exercise, supplementation and an increase in water consumption. Try these before shooting some chemical into your veins. Also, fifty sessions can get very costly and at three hours or so per session, it will eat up your time clock very quickly.

There have been many cases of bad, long-term reactions and

it's not worth the risk unless you absolutely need it. Enough said on this. If you disagree then please research this subject before trying it.

Meditation

Meditation is a deliberate attempt at suspending your thought process with the intent to relax and ease your mind; not to be confused with mediation, which is a deliberate attempt to ease the outflow of your pocketbook. (If you have used the services of a mediator, then you have kept more of your money out of the hands of an attorney and like meditation, have lightened your emotional burden as well.)

Where would we be without mentioning meditation as a valid alternative therapy? It is as old as dirt and has been used for a variety of ailments for thousands of years including anxiety, depression, high blood pressure, chronic pain, asthma, emphysema, PMS and of course, stress. Still, this ancient form of relaxation is fairly new to the United States, not having much exposure before the middle of the twentieth century.

There are three basic types of meditation used. *Transcendental Meditation* involves the repetition of a sound, called a mantra, while in a traditional meditation position or sitting up in a straight back chair. *Breath Meditation,* as the name implies, utilizes the process of inhaling and exhaling at a conscious and deliberate pace. And a Buddhist form called *mindfulness meditation,* or vipassana, concentrates on the present moment, many times doing a sort of body scan that directs your level of consciousness to the different parts of your body, moving up or down depending on where you began.

Regardless of the form that you use, meditation should be a powerful tool in your battle to get and stay healthy. It just works. It does lower your blood pressure, it does relax you, it can relieve chronic pain, and it **will** lower your heart rate. On top of those benefits, meditation helps lower the production of the stress hormones noradrenaline and cortisol, which, by themselves will help you live longer. The best part? You can teach yourself for the cost of a CD, tape, or even a book and then use it the rest of your life to maintain your sanity in this crazy world. You have now and will have in the future enough stress triggers in your personal environment that deserves some of your time and effort. Meditating twice a day, if you can manage that, for fifteen minutes at a time will do you a world of good.

Meditation is now mainstream: 1.5 million people in the U.S. practice transcendental meditation, 6,000 of them are physicians. Even the National Institute of Health is getting into the act by giving an $8 million grant to a college in Iowa to study this and other natural-healing techniques. (Don't tell the pharmaceutical companies or they'll try and find a drug to induce the relaxed state that meditation provides. Oh, yeah. They already have one. It's called Valium.) Many doctors prescribe meditation (not Valium) to their patients and countless studies have shown the benefit of relaxing through meditation.

In over a third of our nation's medical schools, alternative medicines and therapies are being taught, so there **is** hope for our health-challenged country. They may not be emphasized at these schools, but at least your doctor will be aware of them and will be able to recommend treatments that may work and discourage some that won't. This is a step in the right direction.

One in three Americans are using some form of alternative medicine, and even though 75% of them won't tell their doctor, the overwhelming demand by you and your fellow Americans is causing the medical community and our politicians to sit up and take notice. There is the Access to Medical Treatment Act before Congress that if passed, would free doctors to suggest non-approved remedies without fear of being sued. This is another step in the correct direction.

As more and more of us seek "another opinion" and alternatives to the stodgy and slow to change Western medical community, the more choices, along with a greater amount of education will be available to us so that we may be able to make better informed decisions about our health. Now if we can only get more of them approved by our insurance companies. . .

Summary

A man completes an extremely thorough physical with his new, primary care physician. After the results of all the lab work were in, the doctor stated that he was doing "fairly well" for his age. A little concerned about the comment, the guy asked him, "Do you think I'll live to be 90?"

The doctor asked, "Well, do you smoke tobacco or drink beer?"

"Oh no," the man replied. "I've never done those."

Then the doc asked, "Do you eat steaks or barbequed ribs?"

"No, I've heard that all red meat is very unhealthy."

"Do you spend a lot of time in the sun, like playing golf?"

Again, the answer was, "No, I don't. I don't want to get skin cancer."

Then the doctor asked, "Do you gamble, drive fast cars, or fool around with women?"

The man stated that he had never done any of those things.

So the doctor looks at him very perplexed and said, "Then why in hell do you want to live to be 90?"

Good point. The punch-line of this joke assumed that the man was having absolutely no fun and that there was no point in extending his life that long.

Are you having fun? Although this program will probably cause you to alter many of your old habits and make some general changes in your life, those changes don't have to be painful, restrictive or boring. One of the main goals is to make you literally feel better. What's not fun about that?

Maybe you don't view regular exercise as a fun activity. Could that be because you haven't really had a regular exercise program before? Maybe you just couldn't get past the momentum change necessary to get you rolling. I'll bet that when you start getting a little comfortable with it and begin to lose weight, your attitude will change in a hurry. The same holds true for clearing your head from smoking, drinking, and excess caffeine or sugar. Buying a new wardrobe can be very exhilarating. There is no better feeling than having new-found energy or sailing through the winter without even once getting sick.

Gradually throwing out your old diet and replacing it with one that will serve to energize you and improve the function of your immune system can be a challenge, but that's the fun part! You'll get a lot more satisfaction out of eating foods that are meant to nourish you than a lot of the junk that presently makes its way through your body. In fact, your body will tell you how it's feeling. Your skin tone will improve, your muscles will firm up, you'll lose inches everywhere and your entire digestive system will finally perform as it should. You may stop loosing hair, your sense of smell and taste will certainly come back and the aches and pains in your joints will subside.

What's wrong with a good night's sleep? Obviously nothing. How about stringing several restful nights in a row? That would be golden to the insomniacs among us. A little less stress in your life will certainly make you feel better. How about a relaxed state of mind, in general? All of the steps in this program will improve the chemistry of your brain helping you to become more balanced . . . not a bad deal.

Bringing more joy into your life can only serve to benefit you immensely and will improve the lives of everyone around you.

As you can see, embarking on this journey is anything but boring or dull. Taking care of your formerly neglected body for the second half of your life produces so many dividends that having fun will be a natural bi-product of the effort that you make. Having your friends and family notice and compliment the changes is a bonus and will surely bring a smile to your face.

I wish you the best of luck on your journey and look forward to seeing you walking through the park . . . in about forty years.

References

American Association of Naturopathic Physicians, *Nature's Pharmacy,* Publications International, 2001

Atkins, Robert C., M.D., *Dr. Atkins' New Diet Revolution,* Avon Books, 1992

Balch, James F., M.D., Balch, Phyllis A., C.N.C., *Prescription for Nutritional Healing,* Avery Publishing Group, 1997

Barefoot, Robert R., *Death By Diet,* Triad Marketing, 2002

Batmanghelidj, F., M.D., *Your Body's Many Cries For Water,* Global Health Solutions, Inc., 1997

Bragg, Paul C., N.D., Ph.D., Bragg, Patricia, N.D., Ph.D., *Water, The Shocking Proof,* Health Science

Bragg, Paul C., N.D., Ph.D., Bragg, Patricia, N.D., Ph.D., *Apple Cider Vinegar,* Health Science

Bricklin, Mark, *The Practical Encyclopedia of Natural Healing,* Penguin Books, 1990

Castleman, Michael, *Blended Medicine,* St. Martin's Press, 2000

Castro, Miranda, *Homeopathic Guide to Stress,* St. Martin's Press, 1996

Charnetski, Carl J., Brennan, Francis X., *Feeling Good is Good For You,* Rodale, Inc., 2001

Cousins, Norman, *Anatomy of an Illness,* Bantam Books, 1981

Feuling, Timothy J., *Chiropractic Works!* Wellness Solutions, 1999

Ford, Norman, *Natural Remedies,* Galahad Books, 1987

Franz, Marion, J., R.D., M.S., *Fast Food Facts,* International Diabetes Center, 1987

Graber, Richard, Gouin, Paul, M.D., *How To Get A Good Night's Sleep,* Chronimed Publishing, 1995

Griffith, H.Winter, M.D., *Complete Guide to Vitamins, Minerals, & Supplements,* Fisher Books

Haas, Robert, M.D., *Eat to Succeed,* Rawson Associates, 1986

Lappe, Marc, *When Antibiotics Fail,* North Atlantic Books, 1995

Ingram, Cass, M.D., *The Cure is in The Cupboard,* Knowledge House, 1997

Lewis, Laura, C.C.N., *52 Ways to Live a Long & Healthy Life,* The Summit Publishing Group, 1993

Mansfield, John M.D., Arthritis, *The Allergy Connection,* Thorsons Publishing Limited, 1990

Mindell, Earl, R. Ph.D., Ph.D., *Earl Mindell's Secret Remedies,* Freeside Books, 1997

Moyer, Ellen, *Vitamins and Minerals,* Wings Books, 1993

Null, Gary Ph.D., *Healing Your Body Naturally,* Wings Books, 1994

Ody, Penelope, *The Complete Medicinal Herbal,* DK Publishing Books, 1993

Ornish, Dean, M.D., *Eat More, Weigh Less,* Harper Collins Publishers, Inc., 2001

Pressman, Alan, M.D., Buff, Sheila, *The Complete Idiot's Guide to Vitamins & Minerals,* Alpha Books, 1995

Page, Linda Rector, N.D., Ph.D., *Healthy Healing,* Healthy Healing Publications, 1997

Roberts, H.J., M.D., *Aspartame, Is It Safe?* The Charles Press Publishers, 1990

Rondberg, Terry A., "Chiropractic First," *The Chiropractic Journal,* 1998

Sosin, Allan, M.D., Jacobs, Beth Ley, Ph.D., *Alpha Lipoic Acid,* Kensington Publishing Corp., 1998

Teitelbaum, Jacob, M.D., *From Fatigued to Fantastic,* Avery Publishing Group, 1996

Van Straten, Michael, *The Good Health Directory,* New Millennium Books, 2000

Weil, Andrew, M.D., *Eating Well For Optimal Health,* Alfred A. Knopf, Inc., 2000

Weil, Andrew, M.D., *Spontaneous Healing,* Fawcett Columbine Books, 1995

Weinberg, Winkler G., M.D., *No Germs Allowed,* Rutgers University Press, 1996

PERIODICALS

Several issues of each of the following publications were used in the compilation of this book.

Alternatives, Dr. David Williams, Mountain Home Publishing

Bottom Line Personal, Martin Edelston, Publisher

Consumer Reports, Consumer Union

Consumer Reports on Health, Consumer Union

Discover, Buena Vista Magazines

Dr. Andrew Weil's Self Healing, Thorne Communications, Inc.

Life Extension, Life Extension Foundation

Men's Health, MaryAnn Bekkedahl, Publisher

Nutrition Action Health Letter, Center For Science in the Public Interest

The John Hopkin's Medical Letter — Health After 50, Medletter Associates

University of California, Berkeley Wellness Letter, University of California, Berkeley

Useful Websites

Alternative Medicine . . . . alternativemedicine.com
Alternative Health News Online. . . . . altmedicine.com
American Academy of Sleep Medicine. . . . . aasmnet.org
American Academy of
Medical Acupuncture . . . . medicalacupuncture.org
American Botanical Council. . . . . herbalgram.org
American Diabetes Association . . . . diabetes.org
American Heart Association. . . . . americanheart.org
American Obesity Association .obesity.org
American Sleep Apnea Association . . . . sleepapnea.org
American Stroke Association . . . . strokeassociation.org
Association for the Study of Dreams . . . . asdreams.org
Arthritis Foundation. . . . . arthritis.org
Best Filters.com . . . . bestfilters.com
Bottom Line Secrets. . . . . bottomlinepersonal.com
Center for Disease Control and Prevention . . . . .cdc.gov
Center For Science in the Public Interest. . . . . cspinet.org
Consumer's Checkbook (ranks hospitals). . . . . checkbook.org
Consumer Lab. . . . . consumerlab.com
Consumer Reports Online . . . . consumerreports.org
Dr. Michael Murray . . . . doctormurray.com
Dr. David Williams. . . . . drdavidwilliams.com
(US) Food and Drug Administration . . . . fda.gov
Fitness Center — American Heart Association . . . . . . justmove.org
The Grain and Salt Society . . . . celtic-salt.com

Health Care Choices. healthcarechoices.org
Health Grades, Inc.-hospital report cards. . . . . healthgrades.com
HealthLink Medical College
(Wisconsin) . . . . healthlink.mcw.edu/index.html
Herb Medicine . . . . herbmed.org
Hospital Profile Consumer Guide. . . . . hospitalprofiles.org
Innerlight Foundation . . . . innerlightfoundation.com
International Obesity Task Force . . . . iotf.org
Joint Commiss on Accreditation of Healthcare org. . . . . . . jcaho.org
Juice Plus+ . . . . juiceplus.com
Lance Armstrong Foundation . . . . laf.org
Life Extension Foundation . . . . lef.org
Lone Star Health.com (HCA). . . . . lonestarhealth.com
The Medem Network . . . . medem.com
Men's Health Magazine . . . . menshealth.com
Narcolepsy Network. . . . . narcolepsynetwork.org
National Sleep Foundation . . . . sleepfoundation.org
New Scientist . . . . newscientist.com
National Institute of Health . . . . nih.gov
Office of the Surgeon General . . . . surgeongeneral.gov
One Life/
American Heart Association. . . . . onelife.americanheart.org
National Center for
Chronic Disease Prevention . . . . . . cdc.gov/nccdphp/dnpa/obesity
Michael J Fox Foundation (Parkinson's) . . . . michaeljfox.com
National Attention Deficit Disorder Association. . . . . add.org
National Center for
Complementary & Alternative Med. . . . . nccam.nih.gov
Reader's Digest — Health . . . . rd.com
Restless Legs Syndrome Foundation. . . . . rls.org
Rx List . . . . rxlist.com
Rx List — Alternatives. . . . . rxlist.com/alternative.htm
Safe Medication.com. . . . . safemedication.com
Sleep info — National Heart, Lung
& Blood Institute rover2.nhlbi.gov/health/public/sleep/
Sleep Medicine . . . . users.cloud9.net/~thorpy

Sleepnet.com . . . . sleepnet.com
Sleep Research Society.org . . . . sleepresearchsociety.org
Sunrise Herb Shoppe . . . . sunherb.com
Supreme Distribution-coral calcium . . . . . . thesupremecalcium.com
Urban Legends and Folklore
(Just for fun!) . . . . urbanlengends.about.com
U.S. Department of Agriculture. . . . . usda.gov
U.S. News and World Report (Hospital study). . . . . usnews.com
Watercure.com. . . . . watercure.com
Water Quality Association . . . . wqa.org
Web MD . . . . webmd.lycos.com
Xtend-Life. . . . . wz.xtend-life.com
Yahoo Health . . . . yahoo.com/health

Index

D

E

F

G

H

I

K

L

M

N

O

P

S

T

U

V

Y

Z

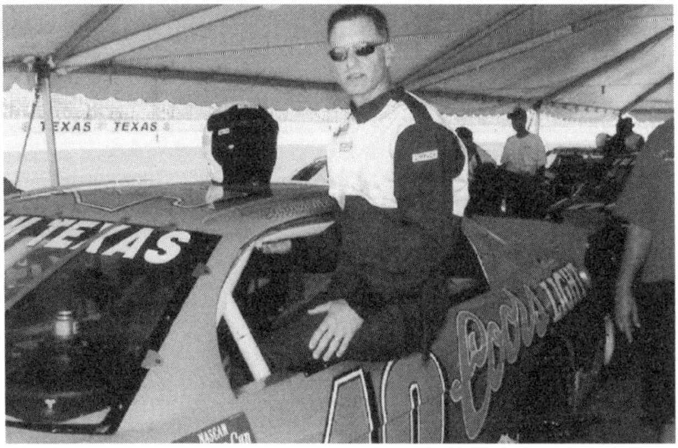

About the Author

"I should have realized right then that my thirties were doomed," Mr. Keith said. On his thirtieth birthday, he tore his left hamstring, and two weeks later his right foot became so infected from a cut while swimming that he was a few days from losing the foot completely. "I was basically limping on one leg and couldn't walk on the other."

The remainder of his fourth decade was filled with many other enjoyable experiences like whiplash from a hard fall while water-skiing that eventually caused excruciating headaches (and a later surgery). He was taking anywhere from fifteen to twenty painkillers daily, virtually every day for the remainder of the decade! He was also skilled at catching every cold or flu that came along (at least two or three a year), many times losing his voice in the process. He managed to tear his other hamstring and endured the trauma from getting married and divorced before the decade was out. The grand finale was being diagnosed with fibromyalgia near the age of forty, which at least explained a lot of his aches and pains. "I was a mess but thought that I was doing all that I could for my health."

Although this book is not about him personally, it is partially the result of his journey back to the good health that he enjoyed early in his life. In the beginning of his investigation, his emphasis was on improving his health, but the last several years were spent further researching and fine-tuning the ten-step process this book is based upon.

Mr. Keith resides in North Texas with his wife and three children.

Do you know someone who could benefit from a copy of this book?

Quantity	Title	Price	Total
	Aging is NOT an Option! *The Baby Boomer's 10-Step Guide to a Long and Healthy Life*	X $ 19.95=	

SUBTOTAL.. $ ______

Texas residents add 8.25% sales tax ______

Shipping:

Normal Delivery (7–10 days) $ 3.95 1st book

Priority Delivery (3–4 days) 5.95 1st book

Add for each additional book 3.00 ______

TOTAL.. $ ______

Note — This form is only for orders within the continental United States. See website for other orders.

Ship To:

Name ______________________________

Address ______________________________

City ____________ **State** ______ **ZIP** ________

Phone (_____ **)** __________ **E-mail** _____ @ __________

Two order choices:

1. Mail this page along with your personal check or money order to the address listed below.
2. Order from our website: agelesspublications.com (credit cards accepted through website)

Thank you for your order. We sincerely hope that your overall health improves from following this program.

AGELESS PUBLICATIONS

P.O. Box 251544, Plano, TX 75025